THE AUTOIMMUNE PALEO COOKBOOK

MICKEY TRESCOTT

NUTRITIONAL THERAPY PRACTITIONER (NTP)

I would like to dedicate this book to those with chronic illness who are looking to bring healing into their lives.

I would also like to dedicate this book to my sister Katie, for being a constant force of youthful energy and support in my life.

AN ALLERGEN-FREE APPROACH TO MANAGING CHRONIC ILLNESS

THE AUTOIMMUNE PALEO COOKBOOK

MICKEY TRESCOTT

NUTRITIONAL THERAPY PRACTITIONER (NTP)

PHOTOGRAPHY BY KYLE JOHNSON

MURDOCH BOOKS

SYDNEY · LONDON

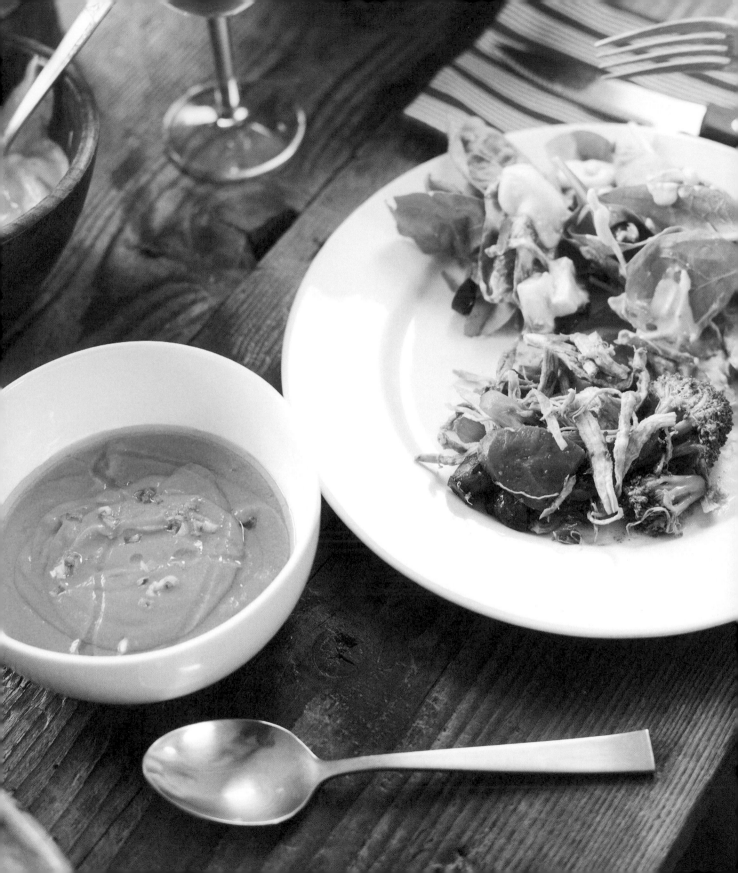

FOREWORD

Diet and lifestyle modifications can be extraordinarily powerful strategies to regulate the immune system, reverse chronic disease, heal the body, and promote overall health. I have a very thorough understanding of the nitty gritty details of how compounds in our foods, the nutrient density of our diets, our hormones, and the 70 trillion probiotic bacteria that live in our guts all interact with our immune system. And I have personal experience with using diet and lifestyle to successfully manage and reverse immune and autoimmune disorders. But I also know that, as powerful as the diet and lifestyle recommendations made in my book, *The Paleo Approach*, are, it can also be overwhelming!

Seeing dramatic improvement in your health can be a great motivator to stick to a restricted diet, but that still doesn't mean that it's easy. And for many, just looking at a list of food 'don'ts' can stimulate the fight-or-flight response. The initial reaction usually includes a mix of panic and trepidation as well as a flood of questions: 'What is there left to eat?' 'How can I possibly make yummy food with such limited ingredients?' 'How will I survive without my favorite comfort foods or convenience foods?' 'How on earth will I entertain company without feeding them bland, weird foods?' And sometimes, we can feel like it's going just fine until we see someone enjoying a piece of cake and then the sense of deprivation hits us like a tonne of bricks.

But you don't need to be intimidated by making big changes to your diet and you don't need to miss out on flavour because *The Autoimmune Paleo Cookbook* has you covered. Simple summary of 'the rules'? Check. Strategies for day-to-day implementation? Check. Meal plans and shopping lists? Check. Amazingly delicious recipes? Check and check!

Mickey Trescott is one of the most talented and creative chefs I know. Her recipes combine flavours in a sophisticated yet simple way, using standard cooking techniques and equipment so that anyone can make them. This book includes a variety of palate-pleasing recipes that comply with the recommendations in *The Paleo Approach*, including: quick everyday meals, elaborate and decadent meals that you could serve to company (and they will never know that they're eating foods belonging to a restricted diet), comfort foods, appetisers, snacks, quick lunches and luscious desserts.

The most important contribution that *The Autoimmune Paleo Cookbook* will make to your life is to reintroduce deliciousness! Being able to eat scrumptious, comforting foods and even enjoy the occasional dessert stops that feeling of 'missing out' in its tracks. It gives you back the contribution that yummy food makes to your quality of life (while also improving your quality of life via a nutritional upgrade). Yes, you can still enjoy good food even while you eat to regulate your immune system and heal your body.

The Autoimmune Paleo Cookbook also helps you get organised with its resources, guides, tips and tricks, meal plans and shopping lists. This takes the guesswork out of what to eat and helps you plan for the week ahead, a strategy that can be essential for success. As much as this cookbook caters to those who follow *The Paleo Approach* to manage immune and autoimmune conditions, this is just plain ol' good food. This book could grace any kitchen bookshelf and the recipes herein could be enjoyed by anyone. And regardless of the reasons you've picked up this book, you will find yourself coming back to these recipes over and over again. So grab a fork and get ready to dig in!

Dr. Sarah Ballantyne, PhD, author of *The Paleo Approach*

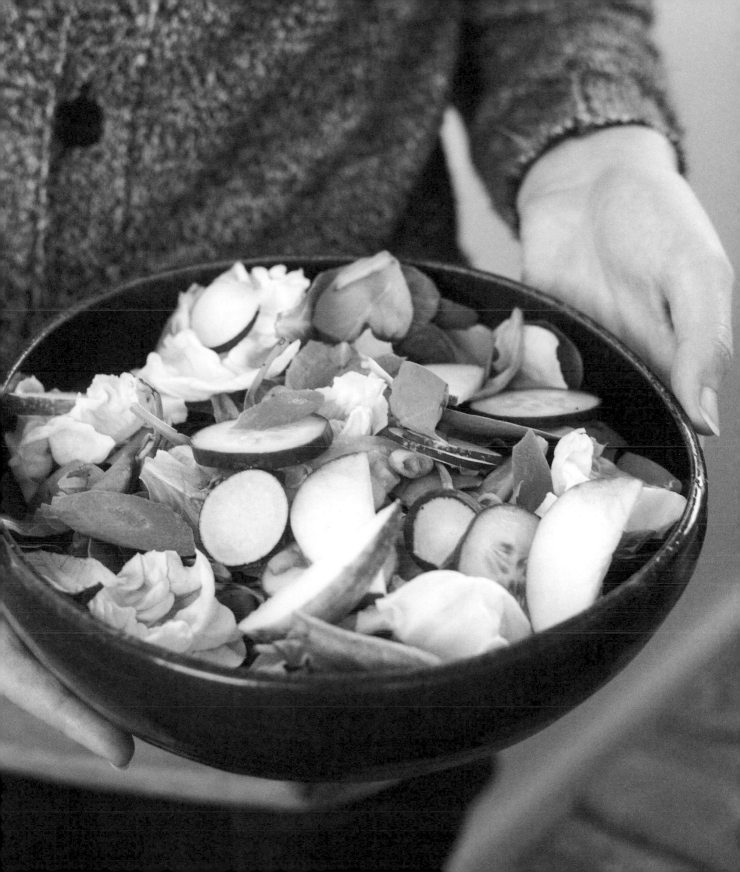

INTRODUCTION

What inspired you to pick up this cookbook? Well, like one in five people in the Western world, you may have been diagnosed with an autoimmune disease, a condition that occurs when the immune system mistakenly attacks one's own tissue.[1] Given that conventional medicine has yet to find a cause or a cure for this condition, you may be left wondering if there is anything you can do to help yourself. Ask your doctor, and you will likely be told that what you eat has nothing to do with your symptoms. However, if you look at how our modern diet has evolved in the last century, with a marked increase in the over-processing of many foods and the emphasis on grains, refined sugar, chemicals, toxins and pesticides, among other elements, it's hard not to see that the food we choose to put into our bodies every day has a direct impact on the rapid increase in chronic illness. What we eat does matter, and just as an improper diet can cause disease, a nourishing one can bring healing—even with a condition as serious as autoimmune disease.

This book is the product of my own personal struggle to find health and vitality using the Autoimmune Protocol—a version of an ancestral diet that removes foods such as grains, beans, dairy, eggs, nuts, seeds and nightshades [a family of plants containing foods like tomatoes, potatoes, eggplants (aubergines) and capsicums]. This diet is designed to heal the gut, or more specifically, the small intestine, which scientists have now pinpointed as a major factor contributing to autoimmune disease.[2]

It was only a short time ago that I felt lost in my own health struggle, not knowing which foods were safe for me to consume or what I could do to manage my condition. I knew I was having food reactions, but I didn't know exactly which foods were causing them. You can imagine then, the excitement I felt after discovering the Autoimmune Protocol and starting to see changes for the better—I finally felt like I had my life back! I used this new-found energy to get back into the kitchen to develop recipes that were free from ingredients that would trigger my symptoms.

In this book I have taken everything I learned on my journey back to health and packaged it so that you can re-create this process for yourself. Implementing the Autoimmune Protocol will help you pinpoint your food allergies and sensitivities as well as gauge how they are affecting your disease. By using this method, you'll find a diet that is most supportive of your individual healing process.

In the first half of the book, you will find a description of exactly what the protocol is, charts outlining what to eat and what to avoid, which foods you can include to promote healing, as well as meal plans and shopping lists to help you transition more quickly. If you're a little more cautious or need more time, I encourage you to start incorporating some of the meals into your routine little by little. Although completely eliminating the problematic foods will have the quickest effect, any move toward a cleaner, more allergen-free diet will help you in the long run.

If there is one takeaway from this book, it is that you do not have to suffer eating a bland, boring diet while eliminating potential food triggers and attempting to regain your health. Despite how daunting it may sound on paper, it is entirely possible to eat varied, flavourful, and interesting meals while on the Autoimmune Protocol, even if some of the most common and convenient foods are removed. Many of these recipes are simple, delicious versions of familiar

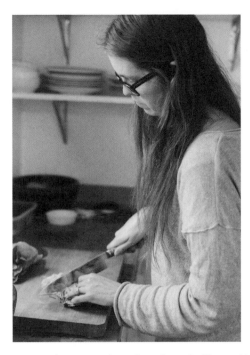

dishes—like 'Spaghetti' and Meatballs (page 282), Chicken Caesar Salad (page 154) or Clam Chowder (page 254). I've also included recipes with ingredients that are a little more out of the ordinary for those who wish to try new flavours, like Moroccan Lamb Stew (page 174), Coconut-Basil Pesto (page 124), Orange-Rosemary Duck (page 220) or Mushroom-Stuffed Cornish Hens (page 223). Armed with these recipes, you can easily create a menu that dinner-party guests will be thrilled to share. Don't be surprised at holiday meals when your allergen-free desserts are consumed faster than the conventional ones!

Another thing to be aware of: eating this way is never going to be as easy as eating a standard Western diet. It takes a lot of discipline, energy and time to successfully make the switch. Even after the transition is made, there will still be an unusual amount of planning and organisation required to keep your kitchen stocked with healing foods at all times. Once you get into a routine, though, tasks like making Solid Cooking Fat (page 42), Fermented Vegetables (page 37), and Bone Broth (page 34), and keeping your freezer stocked full of free-range meats and emergency meals becomes easier. Your kitchen starts to have an ebb and flow; one day you bottle kombucha and roast a chicken, the next you make some broth with the bones. While in the beginning you may need to follow a strict plan and commit everything to paper, you might be surprised when you no longer have to obsess over the details; maintaining the diet becomes routine.

If you are anything like I was at the time I discovered the Autoimmune Protocol, you may be in poor health and without ample time or energy to cook. For those in this circumstance, I've done my best to include simple one-pot meals that can be prepared ahead and used when you need a quick meal. Most of the soups, like Beetroot and Fennel Soup (page 157), Carrot-Ginger Soup (page 157), Classic Chicken Soup (page 160) and Under the Weather Soup (page 172) can be cooked as a double batch and frozen in portion-size containers. Shredded Chicken Breast (page 208) and Shredded Roast Beef (page 256) can be also be cooked in quantity and used to create tasty meals during the week. If you can, recruit willing friends and family members to help you keep healthy food on hand. Once you regain some of your strength and energy, you'll be able to branch out into recipes that require more preparation.

Lastly, on page 302 you will find a section devoted to resources helpful to anyone searching for more information on diet and autoimmunity. There are books and websites on ancestral nutrition, autoimmune disease and digestion that make excellent supplements to the information presented here. I have also included links to resources to help you track down good-quality food, as well as links to help you find practitioners who can help guide you on your path to better health.

MY STORY

In my mid-twenties, following the investigation of some growing health concerns, I was diagnosed with two conditions: Hashimoto's disease (an autoimmune disease that targets the thyroid gland) and Coeliac disease (an autoimmune disease that targets the small intestine). Prior to this experience, I barely knew what an autoimmune disease was, and only knew of a friend-of-a-friend who had one. While I had previously been an active, healthy person, my condition declined rather quickly, until I was unable to work or do any of the activities that I had previously loved—like cycling, rock climbing and running. I sought the help of both conventional and alternative medicines, neither of which had any effective options for me. After months of resting, waiting and further testing, I still didn't have any answers. It was then that I embarked on my own search for healing.

I have always been a believer in food as medicine. Ten years prior, while in college, I experimented with veganism, which resulted in many initial health benefits—the best of which was the disappearance of my severe asthma. I later found out that this condition stemmed from a serious dairy allergy that had been misdiagnosed as asthma in childhood. It was then that I learned how to cook, and I eliminated all processed foods from my diet. While I felt great when I first adopted this diet, after a couple of years I started having some new health concerns: low energy, hair loss and fatigue. When I went to the doctor, I discovered that I was suffering from vitamin deficiencies and would need to rely on supplements to keep my levels up. I thought that these vitamins were all I needed to keep me healthy, but over the years I noticed a steady decline in my energy level and overall health.

By the time I was diagnosed with my autoimmune conditions, I was struggling to get through each day, and relying heavily on caffeine and sugar. After my crash, I asked all of the doctors I saw what they thought of my vegan diet—I wanted to know if it could be one of the reasons I wasn't recovering. They reassured me that a low-fat, plant-based diet with proper supplementation was excellent for my condition. Despite their advice, I was getting worse with every passing month. I tried raw food diets and more supplements, as well as cleanses, some of which further weakened my condition and made me more ill.

In an act of desperation, I decided to entertain the thought that maybe the way I was eating was not optimal for my body. It was from this place that I began to research the connection between diet and autoimmune disease. Through testimonials of those who had healed from chronic health issues, I discovered the concept of the ancestral, or paleo, style of eating. What I found was the notion that a nourishing diet that included the foods of our ancestors and excluded modern convenience products was ideal for maximum healing. I immediately cut out the grains and beans I had been living off of, and slowly started introducing free-range meats, eggs, and wild-caught fish into my diet. I started eating organ meats like liver and soups made with bone broth. After making these changes, I was quickly relieved of the worst of my coldness and fatigue. This encouraged me to believe I was on the right track, although I knew there were still some foods in my diet holding me back from restoring my health.

As I continued my research, I found the work of Dr. Datis Kharrazian, who advocates for a specific diet to heal the gut for those with autoimmune disease.[3] Around the same time, I also discovered that many of the leaders in the ancestral health movement, like Robb Wolf, were advocating a similar approach called the Autoimmune Protocol.[4] All of these experts were basing their recommendations on research in the scientific literature that linked autoimmune disease to gut health. It was apparent that there were additional foods that could be problematic for those with autoimmune disease. This made sense to me, as I had found some success with my diet change but knew that I was still having trouble with certain foods—it was just a matter of pinpointing which ones. All of these sources were leading me in the direction of trying an elimination diet to find out which specific foods I was sensitive to.

I decided to try the Autoimmune Protocol for a few months. Initially, it did not go well. I was tortured by how few foods I could have, and I did not experience the immediate benefits that I had heard of others experiencing. After a few failed starts, I managed to stick with it, and after a few months I felt a shift in my energy. I attempted to reintroduce foods, and my efforts were met with a crashing return of symptoms. It was here that I decided to commit to the Autoimmune Protocol long term, and I continued to see benefits with every passing month. I also started to dig deeper into making lifestyle changes in order to be more gentle on myself and give my body the rest it needed to heal. After another few months of sticking to my plan, I was my healthy, vibrant self once again.

Although it was not the only factor that contributed to my recovery, finding the Autoimmune Protocol and eliminating my food triggers was an incredibly powerful piece of the healing journey. Along with changing my diet, I enlisted the help of a functional medicine practitioner—a doctor who specialises in treating patients as a whole, from a perspective of health instead of disease. I also made the lifestyle modifications recommended by those in the ancestral health community—mainly stress management, sleep, and movement. In order to be successful, I believe a multi-faceted approach such as this gives the best results.

It has been years since my original transition to the Autoimmune Protocol, and although I have been able to incorporate many of the 'foods to avoid' into my diet on a somewhat regular basis, I always return to the stricter protocol in periods of illness or stress. At one point, I struggled with feeling sorry for myself because I realised that I wouldn't be eating certain foods ever again, and would always mistrust the food prepared at restaurants. Now, if anything, I am overjoyed that I found out what works for me, and I am constantly thinking of new ways to prepare safe foods that are creative and flavourful, and that I can share with those I love. Instead of eating out, I enjoy cooking and collaborating with my friends, both those with food allergies and without. Even though this has been a long road, I am forever grateful for the ability to learn how certain foods negatively affect my body, and how other foods bring nourishment and vitality into my life.

THE AUTOIMMUNE
PROTOCOL

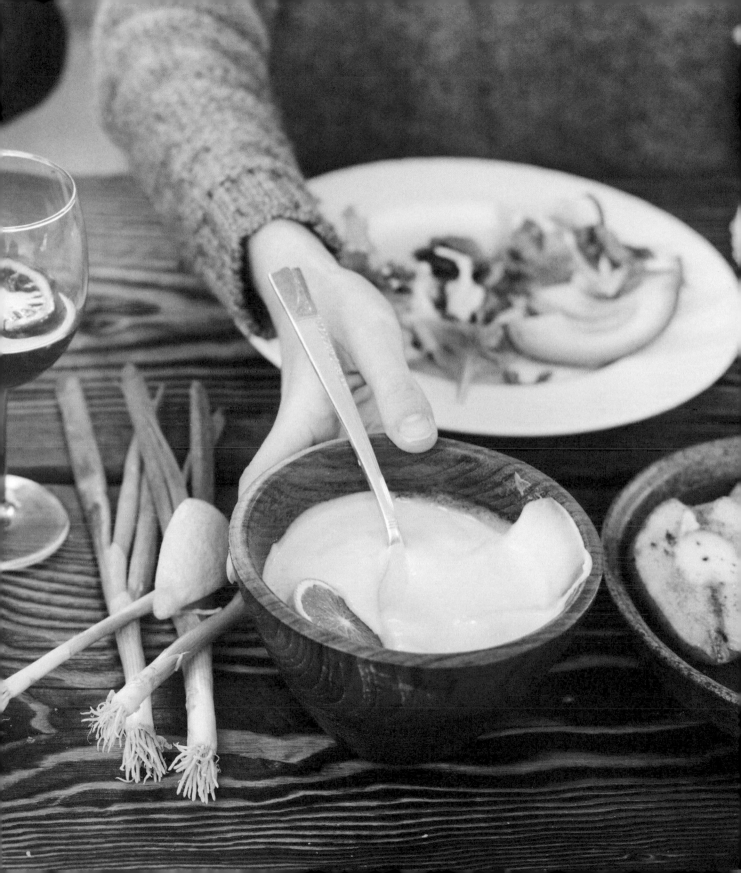

ANCESTRAL DIETS EXPLAINED

Before delving into the specifics of the dietary modifications that help those of us with autoimmune disease, I must explain the ancestral health movement. In the last few years there have been a growing number of health experts, doctors and researchers advocating a new way of eating in order to address the growing health concerns of our modern society—and their answer, in a nutshell, is to eat like our ancestors. How that is defined exactly is up to each advocate and their respective followers, but they all agree that modern foods like grains, beans, refined sugar, vegetable oils and food chemicals are out. In addition to excluding these modern foods, there is also emphasis on adding high-quality animal foods that were available to our ancestors: free-range meats, wild-caught fish, as well as making use of the 'odd bits' like bones and organ meats.[5]

Through eating this way, a growing number of people have found a path to better health and vitality, whether it be better sleep, weight loss, improved digestion, mood or increased energy. Some of the most compelling stories coming out of this movement are the reports of those who suffered for years with chronic health issues that have now been resolved. When the body is given whole, natural foods, free from processing, chemicals and toxins, it enables the natural processes we all have within us to detoxify and heal.

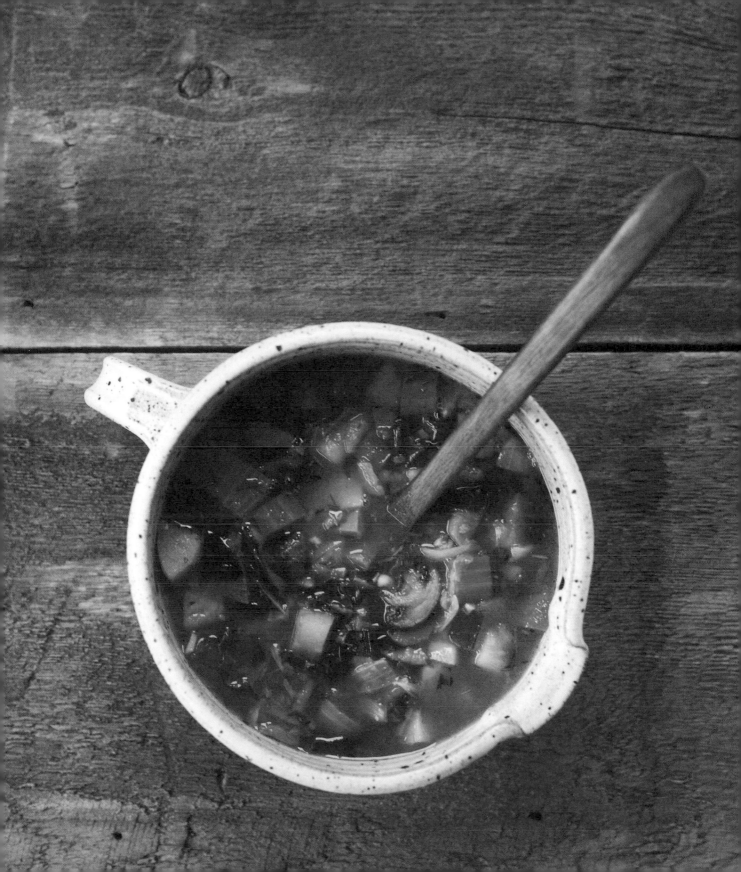

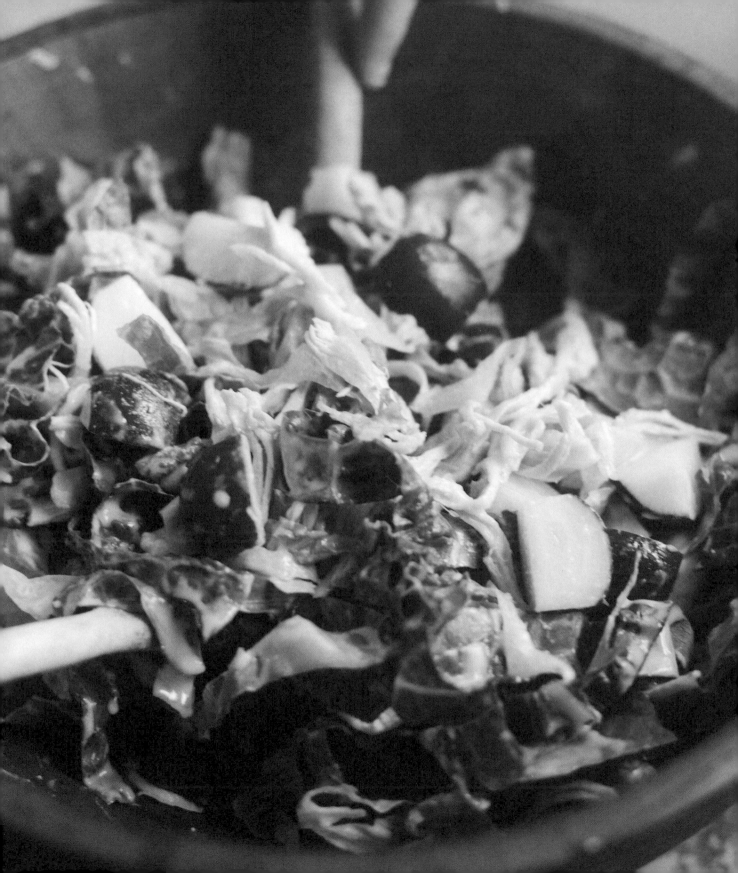

WHAT IS THE AUTOIMMUNE PROTOCOL?

Although eating like our ancestors can be quite powerful at reversing a number of health conditions, it has been recommended by experts in the community that those with autoimmune diseases make further restrictions, at least until the condition is put into remission. The Autoimmune Protocol, also known as the Paleo Approach, is the variation that has been recommended for those with autoimmune conditions.[6] While most ancestral diets avoid grains, beans, legumes, and dairy, the Autoimmune Protocol also removes eggs, nuts, seeds, and nightshade vegetables (such as tomatoes and capsicums—more on that later), food chemicals (like thickeners and alternative sweeteners) and over-the-counter medications like NSAIDs (such as ibuprofen). In addition to removing of all of these products, there is an emphasis placed on replacing them with the highest quality, most nutrient-dense foods available: free-range meats, wild-caught fish, organ meats, bone broth, fermented foods and a colourful array of fruits and vegetables.[7]

Sarah Ballantyne, author of *The Paleo Approach*, has done the most thorough research on the subject, and this book follows her version of the protocol. In addition to dietary modifications, there are many important lifestyle changes that are integral to healing from autoimmune disease that are covered in Sarah's book: increasing sleep, lessening stress, increasing movement and optimising sun exposure.

WHY DOES IT WORK?

The main premise of the Autoimmune Protocol is that it is designed to help heal the gut from both intestinal permeability (otherwise known as 'leaky gut') as well as dysbiosis, both of which have been shown to be present in those with autoimmune disease.[8] Leaky gut occurs when the tight junctions of the cells lining the small intestine become more permeable, letting undigested food, toxins and pathogens into the body, triggering the immune system.[9] Dysbiosis is an imbalance of gut flora (the microorganisms that live in the digestive tract), leading to overgrowths or deficiencies of certain species.[10] Research has shown that the foods and substances avoided on the Autoimmune Protocol contribute to both of these conditions. By removing them from the diet, the gut lining is then able to heal, and proper flora balance can be established. This almost always results in a lessening of symptoms and healing for those facing autoimmune disease.[11]

FOODS TO AVOID

GRAINS

amaranth
barley
buckwheat
burghul
corn
farro
kamut
millet
oats
quinoa
rice
rye
sorghum
spelt
teff
triticale
wheat
wild rice

NUTS

almond
brazil
cashew
cocoa
coffee
hazelnut
macadamia
pecan
pine nut
pistachio
walnut

BEANS + LEGUMES

adzuki beans
black beans
black-eyed peas
broad beans
chickpeas
haricot beans
kidney beans
lentils
lima beans
mung beans
peanuts
soybeans
white beans

SEEDS

anise
canola
caraway
chia
coriander
cumin
fennel seed
fenugreek
flax
hemp
mustard
nutmeg
poppy
pumpkin
sesame
sunflower

EGGS

chicken eggs
duck eggs
goose eggs
quail eggs

DAIRY

butter
buttermilk
casein
cheese
condensed milk
cottage cheese
cream
cream cheese
evaporated milk
frozen yoghurt
ghee
goat's cheese
goat's milk
ice cream
kefir
milk
sheep's milk
sour cream
whey
whey protein
whipped cream
yoghurt

NIGHTSHADES

capsicum
cayenne pepper
chili pepper
chipotle chili pepper
eggplant (aubergine)
goji berry
habanero pepper
jalepeño pepper
paprika
physalis
poblano pepper
potato
tobacco
tomatillo
tomato

OTHER

alcohol
alternative sweeteners
emulsifiers
food additives
food chemicals
NSAIDs (aspirin,
   ibuprofen, naproxen)
stevia
thickeners

FOODS TO INCLUDE

VEGETABLES

artichoke
asparagus
bok choi
broccoli
brussels sprouts
butternut squash
cabbage
cauliflower
celery
chard
courgette (zucchini)
cucumber
fennel
kale
leek
lettuce
mange tout
mushroom
pumpkin
rhubarb
rocket
spinach
spring greens
summer squash
watercress
winter squash

FATS

animal fat
avocado oil
coconut oil
duck fat
lard
olive oil
palm oil
tallow

ROOTS

beetroot
carrot
celeriac
jicama
onion
parsnip
radish
shallot
swede
sweet potato
turnip
yam

MEATS

beef
buffalo
chicken
duck
fish
lamb
pork
rabbit
shellfish
turkey
venison

OFFAL

bone broth
gizzards
heart
kidney
liver
tongue

FRUIT

apple
apricot
avocado
banana
blackberry
blueberry
cantaloupe
cherry
clementine
coconut
date
fig
grape
grapefruit
guava
honeydew
kiwi
lemon
lime
mango
nectarine
orange
papaya
peach
pear
persimmon
pineapple
plum
pomegranate
raspberry
strawberry
tangerine
watermelon

HERBS

basil
bay leaves
chamomile
chives
coriander
dill
lavender
lemongrass
marjoram
mint
parsley
peppermint
rosemary
sage
spearmint
tarragon
thyme

SPICES

cinnamon
cloves
garlic
ginger
saffron
sea salt
turmeric

PANTRY

apple cider vinegar
anchovies
arrowroot flour/
    starch
coconut aminos
coconut flakes
    (unsweetened)
coconut flour
coconut vinegar
desiccated coconut
    (unsweetened)
olives
oysters
salmon
sardines
tea
tuna
ume plum vinegar

OCCASIONAL SWEETENERS

dates
dried fruit
honey
maple syrup
treacle

FERMENTS

fermented vegetables
    (carrots,
    beetroots and
    other vegetables)
kombucha
sauerkraut
water kefir

THE ARGUMENT FOR NUTRIENT DENSITY

While avoiding foods that contribute to leaky gut and dysbiosis are an important part of the protocol, equally important is increasing the amount of nutrient-dense foods. These nutrients are desperately needed by the body to heal the gut and nourish the body. It may seem like the elimination of so many foods from the diet would result in nutrient deficiencies, but that is hardly the case—this way of eating is much more nutrient-dense than the standard Western diet and is perfectly healthy to continue long term. It is particularly high in nutrients needed for healing and recovery: the fat-soluble vitamins A and D, the B vitamins, omega-3 fatty acids, as well as other minerals and nutrients like zinc, selenium, carotenoids and sulphur. Given this, in order to be successful you must diligently seek out the most nutrient-dense foods and include them in your diet on a regular basis.

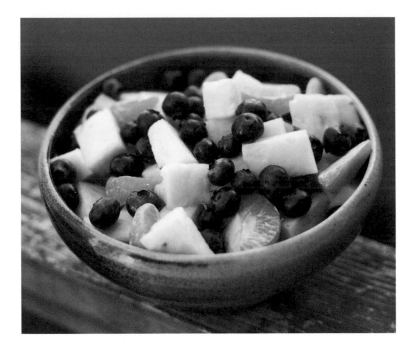

This means eating a varied diet that includes organ meats like liver and kidney, fatty fish and shellfish, seaweed, fermented foods and tonnes of colourful fruits and vegetables. Do not ignore this piece of the protocol! A lot of these foods are not common or palatable for many, but they were an integral part of our ancestors' diets. I would encourage you to step out of your comfort zone and make an effort to include these foods in order to bring more of these nutrients into your diet.

Here is a list of important nutrients and some of the Autoimmune Protocol compliant foods they are found in.[12] This list is by no means exhaustive, but you can see why it is of the utmost importance to include certain foods in your diet (dare I mention liver and fatty fish?).

FAT-SOLUBLE VITAMINS

Vitamin A: Liver and fish liver oil (for retinol) and yellow-orange vegetables (for beta carotene, which is a precursor to vitamin A).

Vitamin D: Liver and fish liver oil, fatty fish and sunlight exposure.

Vitamin E: Red palm oil, coconut oil, olive oil and green leafy vegetables.

Vitamin K: Organ meats, cruciferous and dark green leafy vegetables, and fermented foods.

OTHER NUTRIENTS

Carotenoids: Colourful vegetables such as carrots, squash, sweet potatoes and beetroots.

Essential Fatty Acids: Fatty fish and fish liver oil, free-range meats and organ meats.

Sulphur: Cruciferous vegetables such as broccoli, kale and cabbage.

WATER-SOLUBLE VITAMINS

B vitamins: Meat and seafood (especially shellfish and organ meats), colourful vegetables and seaweed.

Vitamin C: Colourful fruits and vegetables, especially citrus and green leafy vegetables.

MINERALS

Calcium: Dark green leafy vegetables, bone broth and sardines.

Copper: Shellfish and liver.

Iodine: Fish, shellfish and seaweed.

Iron: Muscle meat, organ meat, fish, shellfish and dark green leafy vegetables.

Magnesium: Dark green leafy vegetables, orange vegetables, bone broth and sardines.

Potassium: Fish, cruciferous and dark green leafy vegetables and orange vegetables.

Selenium: Fish, shellfish, organ meats and muscle meats.

Zinc: Shellfish, organ meats, muscle meats and green leafy vegetables.

OTHER FACTORS

In addition to removing specific foods and increasing the overall nutrient density of your diet, there are other factors that can help you on your road to recovery. Although this book is mostly about the dietary aspect of healing, it would be incomplete without the acknowledgement of some of the lifestyle factors that are crucial for recovering your health. For more information about these, and other steps you can take to help yourself through this process, I highly recommend checking out Sarah Ballantyne's incredible book, *The Paleo Approach*, where she goes into more detail about these important lifestyle changes.

· **Sleep:** Make sure you are sleeping well—this is essential for healing and allowing your body to restore itself. Aim for at least eight hours of uninterrupted sleep per night—more if you can manage it.

· **Stress management:** Engage in at least one activity aimed at reducing your stress level every day, whether it be meditation, walking, taking a bath or anything else that helps you to relax.

· **Movement:** Make an effort to do one movement-based activity every day. This could be gentle exercise like yoga, qigong or walking, or a more intense activity like bike riding, running or hiking.

· **Sunlight exposure:** It is very important to get sunlight exposure on some part of your body (it could just be your face and arms) for 20 minutes every day. This stimulates your body's production of vitamin D, which is extremely important to the healing process.

In addition to these lifestyle factors, finding a practitioner trained in functional medicine can be an invaluable part of monitoring your progress with testing as well as making individual supplement recommendations. Be sure to visit the resources section (page 302) to find practitioners who integrate dietary approaches into their practices.

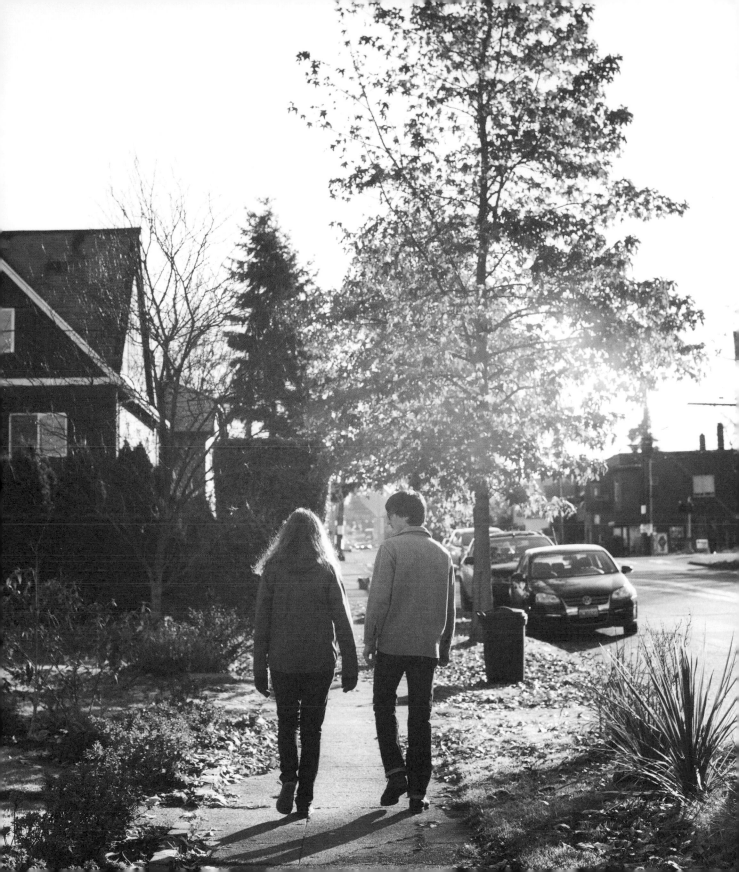

REINTRODUCING FOODS

At some point after implementing the Autoimmune Protocol, a person should start to see improvement (and in some cases, depending on the original condition, even remission). This usually takes at least a month, but can take up to a few months or more of eating strictly according to the protocol. Once a person starts to see a measurable improvement, it is up to them whether they want to play it safe and continue on (in an effort to experience deeper healing), or if they want to try to reintroduce some of the 'safer', disallowed foods. The point at which a person arrives at the place where reintroductions are possible is highly individual, and there is no way to tell how long it will be until you try.

That being said, it is extremely important *not* to start reintroducing foods until you see a *measurable* improvement in your symptoms. If you start too soon, you will have nothing to gauge your reaction against. I encourage you to stay on the Autoimmune Protocol as long as you can, letting yourself heal as much as possible before reintroducing foods. When it comes time for reintroductions, it will be absolutely clear which foods are affecting you. If you've been on the Autoimmune Protocol for a few months with no improvements, it may be appropriate to enlist the assistance of a functional medicine practitioner to help with further testing.

The protocol for reintroductions, as outlined by Sarah Ballantyne in *The Paleo Approach*, is as follows:

1. Pick a food to challenge and get ready to eat it a couple of times in one day.
2. Eat the food for the first time, only having a nibble. Wait 15 minutes, and if you don't have any symptoms, take a small bite, a little larger than the last.
3. Wait another 15 minutes, and if you still don't have any symptoms, take another bite, again slightly larger.
4. Wait two-to-three hours, watching to see if any symptoms appear.
5. Next, eat an average quantity of the food, either by itself of as a part of a meal.
6. Watch your symptoms for three-to-seven days afterwards, being sure to avoid the food you reintroduced as well as not reintroducing any other foods.
7. You may incorporate the food into your diet if you have no symptoms during this whole process.

When you reintroduce a food, you are looking for *any* type of reaction to that food. It could be the return or worsening of your autoimmune symptoms: digestive changes or upset, headaches, dizziness, problems with energy or sleep, joint or muscle pain, skin changes like rashes or acne, or even changes in mood. Reactions can be immediate, or they could show up a day or two after the fact. If you think your reaction to a certain food is a coincidence with some other external factor, like illness or stress, wait until you recover and reintroduce again.

I like to keep a journal for tracking food reintroductions. The more information you are able to track, the better. It's a good idea to plan your reintroductions for a time when you are feeling good and not under a lot of stress. This way you have more energy to devote to assessing your condition and tracking the process, and you will know that the symptoms you are experiencing are from the foods and not just from other influences.

According to Sarah Ballantyne, foods should be reintroduced in stages. Those in stage 1 have the highest chance of being tolerated, while those in stage 4 have the least. While you should be careful to only introduce foods one at a time, you should also attempt to try all of the foods in stage 1 before moving on to stage 2. This means your first food reintroductions should be along the lines of egg yolks and seed spices, not tomatoes or milk (sorry!). Here are the stages, as outlined in *The Paleo Approach*:

STAGE 1:

Egg yolks
Legumes with edible pods
Fruit and berry-based spices
Seed-based spices
Seed and nut oils
Ghee from grass-fed dairy

STAGE 2:

Seeds
Nuts (except cashews and pistachios)
Cocoa or chocolate
Egg whites
Butter from grass-fed dairy
Alcohol (in small quantities)

STAGE 3:

Cashews and pistachios
Eggplants (aubergines)
Capsicums
Paprika
Coffee
Raw cream from grass-fed dairy
Fermented raw dairy (yoghurt and kefir)
   from grass-fed dairy

STAGE 4:

Other dairy products (whole milk and
   cheese from grass-fed dairy)
Chili peppers
Tomatoes
Potatoes
Other nightshades and nightshade spices
Alcohol (in larger quantities)
White rice
Traditionally prepared legumes
   (soaked and fermented)
Traditionally prepared gluten-free grains
   (soaked and fermented)
Foods you have a history of severe reaction to
Foods you are allergic to

Once you begin reintroducing foods and learning how to gauge your reactions to them, you will start to piece together a safe diet that best manages your condition. While a negative reaction to a food can be discouraging, don't discount that you may be able to tolerate that food a few months down the line as your body continues to heal. My advice is to be cautious, take it slow and, when in doubt, leave it out. Over time, you will learn to better listen to your body's language as it tells you how to discern which foods are promoting health and which ones are slowing your progress.

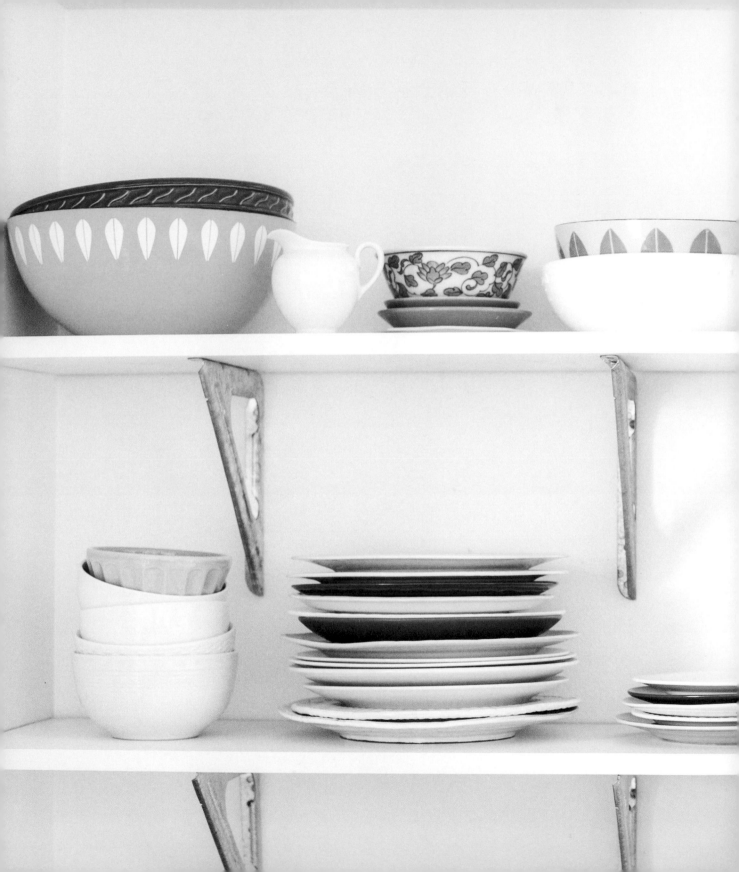

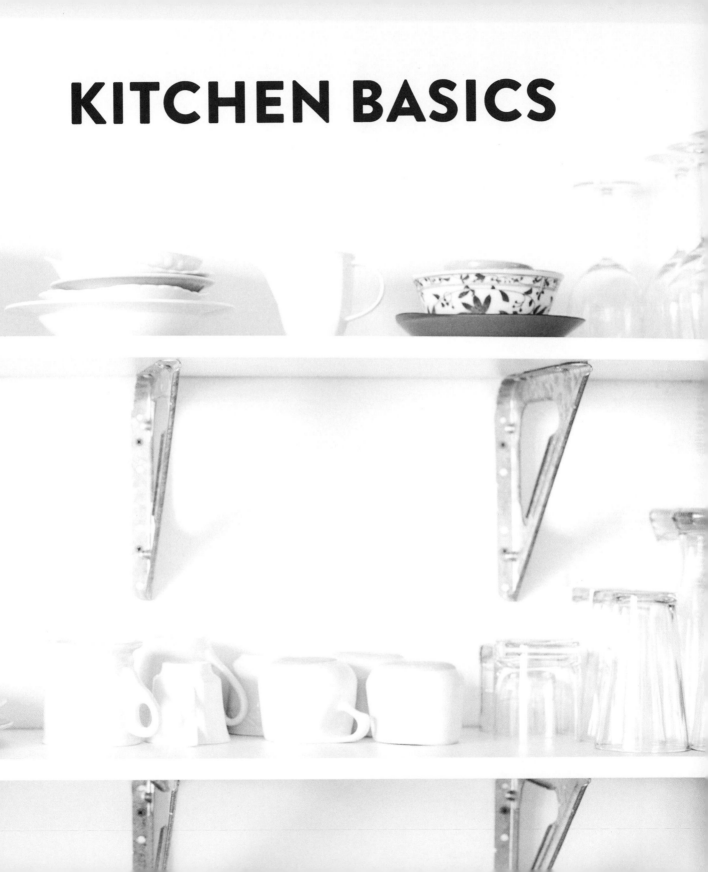

KITCHEN BASICS

STOCKING YOUR KITCHEN
WITH REAL FOODS

So you've been convinced to try the Autoimmune Protocol with the aim of bringing your body back to health. That is awesome! But how do you convert your kitchen from a place of constant temptation to one that promotes your healing journey?

The first step is to remove all the most obvious foods that will be detrimental to your progress. This means that all items containing gluten, plus processed foods, refined sugar, treats, snack foods, convenience foods and the like should be removed from your cupboards. If you still have family members who wish to eat these foods, ask them if they would be willing to store them where they won't be encountered in your daily routine (and try to convince them that they shouldn't be eating processed food and sugar anyway!). You do not need to remove everything excluded on the Autoimmune Protocol—things like nuts, seeds and spices are fine to keep around until you are ready to try reintroductions. It is very important, however, to make sure you get rid of any snacks or quick, easy, convenience foods you could access at a time of weakness during your elimination diet. Examine the ingredients of everything in your cupboards carefully.

Once you have your pantry and cupboards clear, it's time to stock them full of foods you *can* have. While the Autoimmune Protocol lends itself to a lot of fresh cooked food and not a lot to easily storable convenience foods, I have given you some ideas of items you can keep in your pantry that are called for in recipes throughout the book. Other foods, like tinned fish, can be useful in case of an emergency when you have no other options available.

Next, you'll want to get into the routine of batch cooking gut-healing foods like Bone Broth (page 34), Fermented Vegetables (page 37), and fermented beverages like Kombucha (page 38) and Water Kefir (page 41). I call for Bone Broth in many of the recipes in this book, and there's a reason for that: it adds gelatin, collagen, minerals and other nutrients that help heal the gut. It can even replace your morning coffee! Fermented foods and beverages are great to consume in order to get a daily dose of probiotics. While you don't *have* to use these recipes, I believe that incorporating them into your diet gives you the best chance of success while on the Autoimmune Protocol.

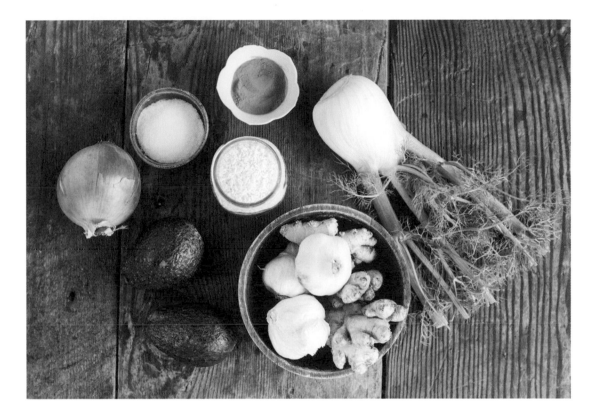

In addition to the gut-healing recipes you will learn, having some other basic recipes in your arsenal will make the task of providing yourself nutritious and varied meals a little easier. Rendering your own fat from free-range animals (page 42) is an inexpensive and healthful way to obtain solid cooking fat to use daily in your kitchen. Also, regularly making batches of Coconut Concentrate (page 45) and Creamy Coconut Milk (page 46) cuts down on the time it takes to prepare recipes that call for these ingredients.

Lastly, I have included a section on which kitchen tools you will find useful for preparing the recipes in this book. While you don't need to go out and purchase any wild appliances, there are some basic tools you will need—after all, you'll be spending a lot of time in the kitchen!

PANTRY ITEMS

· Anchovies – Use to flavour dressings and to add to salads. Check the ingredients to ensure they are packed in olive oil and have no other additives.

· Arrowroot flour/starch – I use arrowroot occasionally as a thickener in some of the recipes in this book. Large bags of it are often less expensive than the tiny bottles you often find in the spice section.

· Avocado oil – A nice oil to have on hand to use in salad dressings and other cold applications. Although I don't call for it in this book, it can replace olive oil in any of the recipes. Purchase a cold-pressed variety, and store it in an opaque bottle away from light and heat, as it oxidises easily.

· Coconut aminos – A product that is similar to soy sauce but made from coconut. Use in Asian-themed dishes to replace soy sauce. If you have trouble sourcing it, check my online resources (page 303).

· Coconut concentrate – A concentrated coconut flesh product (also known as coconut cream, coconut butter or coconut 'manna') that is solid at room temperature. It can be used to make dressings, thicken sauces and stews or may be eaten by itself. I have included a recipe to make it (page 45), but it can also be purchased commercially.

· Coconut crystals – Sugar made from the evaporated syrup from coconut trees. I would use this sparingly—I only call for it in one recipe in the book (Apple-Cranberry Crumble, page 299).

· Coconut flour – Flour made from the dried flesh of coconuts. I use this in a couple of the dessert recipes in this book.

· Coconut milk – Use to thicken soups and stews, to add to smoothies, or to drink by itself. Try to find a brand without non-compliant thickeners, like guar gum.

· Coconut oil – An excellent solid cooking fat to use for cooking and baking. Look for products that are not processed with heat or chemicals, if possible.

· Dried fruit – Nice to have on hand for the occasional sweet treat or to add to a dessert recipe. I like having dates, raisins, currants and dried apricots handy.

· Dried herbs and spices – Bay leaves and ground spices like turmeric, cinnamon, ginger and cloves are all seasonings that you should have on hand. If you don't have a source of fresh herbs like thyme, rosemary, sage, oregano, basil or tarragon, it might be nice to keep a small stock of those in their dried form.

· Extra-virgin olive oil – An excellent oil for using cold, like adding to already-cooked fish or salad dressings. Choose a high-quality, pure oil (free from additives) that is sold in an opaque bottle. Be sure to store away from light and heat, as it oxidises easily.

· Gelatin – Although I don't call for it in the book, having some gelatin (from grass-fed animals) is nice if you can't source bones for making broth. It can also be used to thicken desserts and to make jelly sweets.

· Honey – I have this on hand to use sparingly when I need just a touch of sweetness. If possible, choose a raw honey local to your area.

· Maple syrup – I like this ingredient because it adds a complex flavour to desserts, although I would recommend not going overboard with sweeteners while on the protocol. Grade B is preferable because it is richer in nutrients.

· Olives – Olives are a common recipe ingredient and are excellent to have on hand for snacks and to add to salads. Be sure to check the label for ingredients other than oil or vinegar, and avoid purchasing any olives in bulk if you are not sure of the ingredients (many places pack them in seed oils and add nightshade spices).

· Sea salt – Sea salt is full of trace minerals and free from anti-caking agents and additives. The type is not as important as its level of processing (the less processed, the better).

· Tapioca flour/starch – I use tapioca as a thickener in a few of the recipes in this book, but some people with severe gluten intolerance may be sensitive to it—in this case use arrowroot instead.

· Tinned seafood – An excellent choice for emergency meals, especially when you're travelling or on the go. Sardines, salmon, tuna, oysters and herring are all favorites. Choose brands that are certified for sustainable fishing practices and that pack their products in BPA-free tins. Be sure to double-check the tin for avoided ingredients like soybean or cottonseed oil.

· Unsweetened desiccated and shredded coconut – These are dried flakes made from the flesh of fresh coconut. Use them as an addition to salads and to make snacks and desserts. They can also be blended to make your own Coconut Concentrate (page 45). Be sure to purchase the full-fat, unsweetened variety. It's nice to have both large- and small-flake varieties on hand.

· Vinegar – Any type of vinegar is acceptable to use on the Autoimmune Protocol, but the label still must be checked for gluten-free status. Some aged vinegars are stored in casks sealed with wheat paste, so if you have a product in mind, it may be a good idea to call the company just to double-check. I like to have apple cider vinegar, ume plum vinegar and coconut vinegar on hand.

GUT-HEALING FOODS

Removing certain foods from the diet is only part of the Autoimmune Protocol; in order to be successful, you must also pay careful attention to increasing the nutrient density and incorporating healing foods into your diet. I am a proponent of consuming fermented foods every day, whether that be eating fermented vegetables or having a probiotic beverage like kombucha or water kefir. In addition to ferments, bone broth is an integral part of healing the gut. It can be enjoyed as a warming beverage in the morning or afternoon instead of coffee, and your body will thank you for all of the healing minerals and nutrients contained within. Even if you don't want to drink it by itself, a large majority of the recipes in this book call for it, so it is something you should always have on hand, either fresh or frozen in advance. Please don't replace this with store-bought broth or stock—it is not the same thing. In many cases, commercial broth contains additives and ingredients that are not included on the Autoimmune Protocol, and is not made from free-range animals.

Bone Broth

Traditionally, humans consumed bone broth as an integral part of soups, stews and sauces made by using large, bone-in pieces of meat. Over time our culture has strayed from using the whole animal in favor of the leanest cuts of meat, without any trace of the odd bits. This is a travesty considering all of the nutrition that can be gleaned from the leftover bones, cartilage, joints and marrow we usually throw away. Thankfully, bone broth has been making a comeback due to its many health benefits. Broth is rich in collagen, which is incredibly useful for maintaining healthy joints, skin and hair, as well as gelatin, which has gut-healing qualities. It is also rich in the minerals that are needed to make bone, which makes it a very restorative and balancing item to include in our diets. Make a batch or two on the weekends and have it available for drinking in the morning instead of coffee, as well as to use in soups, stews and sauces.

Fermented Vegetables

Many traditional cultures used fermentation as a way to preserve foods for long periods of time without the need for canning or refrigeration. During the process of lacto-fermentation, beneficial bacteria break down the food to make it richer in enzymes and nutrients. These beneficial bacteria promote the growth of healthy gut flora in our intestines and are an integral component of a healing diet. Including a scoop of fermented vegetables every morning with breakfast is a great way to get some of this probiotic food on a regular basis.

Probiotic Beverages

Both kombucha and water kefir are fermented beverages that are made from starter cultures, although they are a little different from each other. Both of them contain probiotics and aid digestion and immune function. While the kombucha contains more acids and enzymes (ideal for aiding digestion), water kefir tends to have more probiotic content. Including one or both is not essential to a gut-healing protocol, but I find them beneficial (and fun to make).

Kitchen Staples

In addition to some store-bought staples I like to have handy in my pantry, there are a few recipes that I like to make on a weekly basis. Since high-quality, rendered animal fat is both costly and hard to find, I believe it is essential to render your own from fat that you source locally. This is the 'solid cooking fat' referenced in many of my recipes, and as you will see from the upcoming section on which fats to cook with, it is essential to do any high-heat cooking with a healthy saturated fat. I also find it preferable to have a couple of different fats available for cooking to add flavour and variety. If you don't have access to quality animal fat in your area, coconut oil and red palm oil are saturated-fat alternatives.

In addition to having a variety of solid cooking fats to choose from, I like to make a couple of staples from coconut products to have handy for recipes. I call for Coconut Concentrate (page 45) as well as Creamy Coconut Milk (page 46) in many of my recipes to get a creamy consistency. It would be wise to include making these items during your weekly batch-cooking routine so that they can be quickly added to meals and recipes during the week.

BONE BROTH

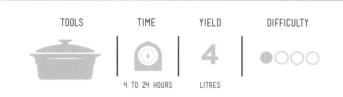

4 TO 24 HOURS   4 LITRES

4 litres filtered water

1 kg (or more) bones from a good source (knuckle and marrow bones work well, but you can use any type of bones)

2 tablespoons apple cider vinegar

1 bay leaf

Stovetop method:

1 Place all ingredients in a large stockpot or slow-cooker and bring to a boil. Lower the heat so the water is barely simmering; cover. Occasionally skim the surface for any scum that may appear during cooking.

2 Cook for at least 8 and up to 24 hours, being sure to check periodically to ensure the broth is still at a bare simmer. The longer you cook your bones, the more rich and nutritious the broth will be.

Pressure Cooker method:

1 Place all ingredients in a pressure cooker, making sure not to exceed the fill line. Lock the lid and place over high heat until the cooker comes to high pressure, then turn down to the lowest setting that will maintain this pressure (you may need to use a flame tamer).

2 Let the broth cook this way for 3 hours, then turn off the heat and let the broth depressurise and cool naturally.

When the broth is finished (using either method):

3 Let cool, then strain and portion the broth into containers for storage. After the liquid is strained, pick through any bones that are still intact and save them to add to the next batch, tossing those that fell apart. (You can usually get a few batches out of larger beef knuckle bones, while chicken bones last only 1 to 2 batches.)

Variation: There are many ways to vary your bone broth, such as browning the bones in the oven before cooking or adding some herbs and spices or vegetables while it is cooking. I like to avoid salting my broth so that it doesn't impact the amount of salt used in recipes. The broth can also be boiled to reduce so that it is concentrated and stored more easily. As you continue to make broth you will get into a flow, and can make it according to your preference. I have added some links to resources on page 303 for further reading on alternate methods as well as the benefits of bone broth.

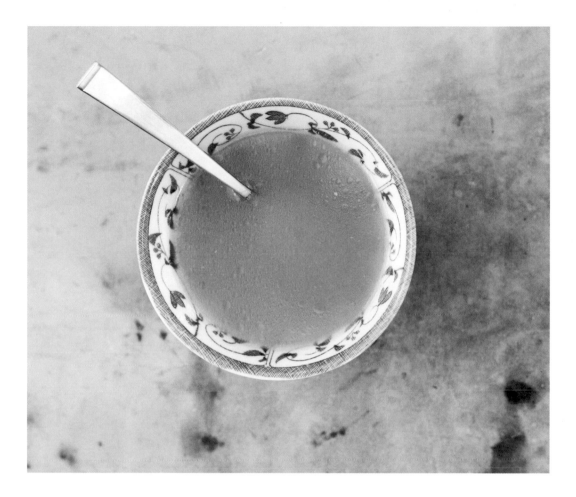

Sourcing Note: Bones should not be expensive or difficult to find. The best source is from a farmer you trust, maybe at a farmers' market or through a local farming co-operative. If you don't have those sources available to you, a lot of health-food stores sell bones from grass-fed meat—be sure to ask the butcher if you don't see any available! Also, you can start a bag in your freezer for storing any bones from the meat you consume—just toss them into the bag and make broth at a later time. Feel free to use any type of bones, even if they have been previously cooked, to make broth; beef, lamb, chicken and turkey all work well.

Storage: Keeps in the refrigerator for a week. Also freezes well.

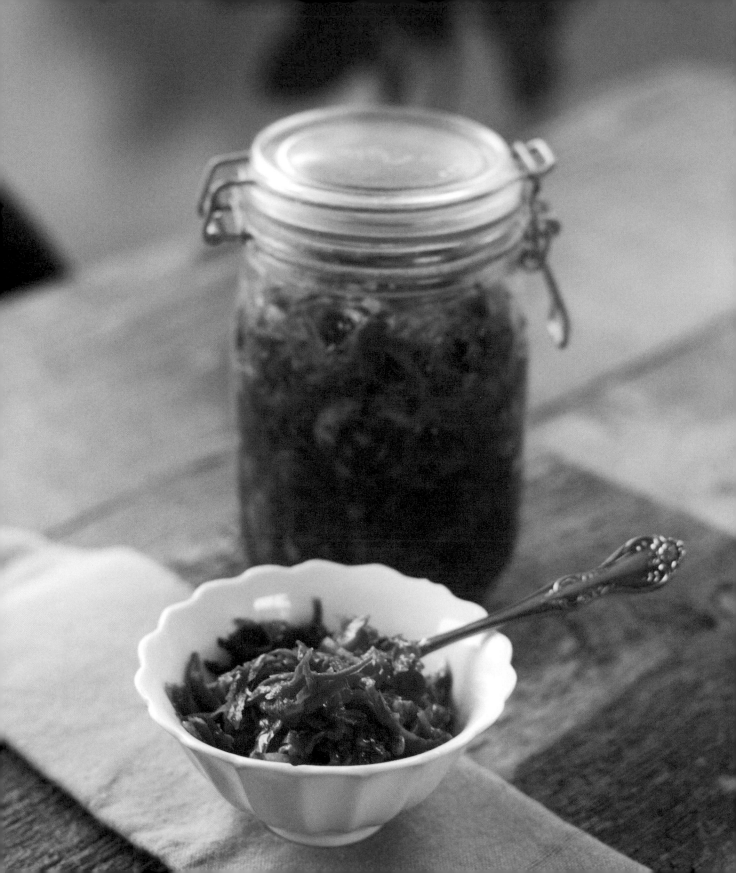

SIMPLE SAUERKRAUT

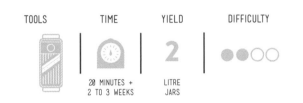

TOOLS	TIME	YIELD	DIFFICULTY
	20 MINUTES + 2 TO 3 WEEKS	2 LITRE JARS	●●○○

2 kg cabbage (about 2 medium heads)
2 tablespoons sea salt

You also need:
2 x 1-litre glass jars with airlocks
Clean fermenting weights or stones
Tamper (optional)

1 Finely shred the cabbage and place it in a bowl in batches, sprinkling each batch with a layer of sea salt. When you are finished with the shredding, use your hands to massage the cabbage well until it breaks down and becomes soft (about 10 minutes). Let the massaged cabbage sit for 10 minutes to let it release its juices.

2 Pack the cabbage very tightly into jars, pushing all of it down until it is completely submerged by its own juices (a tamper is helpful here). Leave about 4 cm head space, and add some additional brine (made by dissolving 1 teaspoon sea salt in 250 ml of water) if there is not enough liquid to fully submerge the cabbage. Place the fermenting stones on top to weigh down the cabbage, tighten the lid and ensure the airlock is installed properly (refer to the instructions that came with your unit, as they can vary). It is possible to ferment without an airlock; be sure to check out some of the online resources on page 303 for further information.

3 Let the cabbage ferment at room temperature for 2 to 3 weeks; during this time, the sauerkraut will bubble a little and intensify in flavour. If any scum appears, remove it with a spoon. Taste it starting at two weeks, and when the taste is to your liking, you can remove the airlock, put a regular lid on the jars and store in the refrigerator.

Variations: The possibilities for varying your fermented vegetables are endless— you can use different types of cabbage, carrots, beetroots, garlic, ginger and many other vegetables in different combinations to make a rich array of tasty probiotic foods. Check the resources on page 303 for links to great websites dedicated to the practice of fermentation.

Storage: The sauerkraut will keep for a few months in the refrigerator.

KOMBUCHA

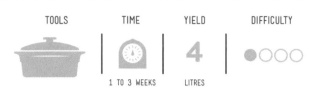

TOOLS	TIME	YIELD	DIFFICULTY
	1 TO 3 WEEKS	4 LITRES	●○○○

4 litres filtered water

5 bags of green tea

220 g granulated sugar (don't use honey or agave here)

1 kombucha starter culture*

250 ml starter liquid (this should either come with the starter culture or be from a previous batch. If you don't have either you can use apple cider vinegar.)

You will also need:

1 x 4-litre glass container

Muslin

Large rubber band

For bottle-fermenting:

Glass jars with lids

Fruit juice

1 Bring the water to a boil, turn off the heat and add the tea bags. Steep for a minute or two and remove.

2 Add the sugar and stir to combine. Let cool completely to room temperature.

3 When the sweetened tea has cooled, pour it into your glass container with the starter culture and starter liquid (don't do this before it is cooled—you will kill your culture!). Cover with a muslin secured with a rubber band and let the jar sit in a dark corner at room temperature (about 20 to 26°C).

4 You can choose to let your culture ferment for at least a week and up to a few weeks, with it getting less sweet and more sour toward the end, as the bacteria eats up most of the sugar. Taste it, and when you like the result, pour most of the kombucha, sparing the culture, into jars and store them in the refrigerator. Leave about 500 ml of liquid in the bottom of the jar to start the next batch. You will also want to remove the new culture that has formed on the top and use it to start another batch, or you could give it to a friend!

Bottle Fermenting: To make your kombucha fizzy, put an 30 to 60 ml of fresh fruit juice in the bottom of a few 1-litre glass jars and fill them to within 2.5 cm of the top of the jars with kombucha. You can use any type of juice you like here—pineapple, grape and pomegranate are some of my favorites. You can also add spices like ginger, turmeric or clove. Screw the lids on tightly and allow the liquid to ferment at room temperature for a couple of days, being sure to open the lids and 'burp' them once a day. When they are finished, put in the refrigerator end enjoy.

*Note: You can find a starter culture (called a scoby) at some health-food stores as well as online, but the best source is to find someone you know locally who can give you a 'baby' from a successful culture. The scoby looks like an opaque, jelly-like glob and should come accompanied by some starter liquid. Once you make your kombucha for the first time, you will end up with an extra scoby to start a double batch or give to a friend!

Storage: Kombucha keeps for a few months in the refrigerator.

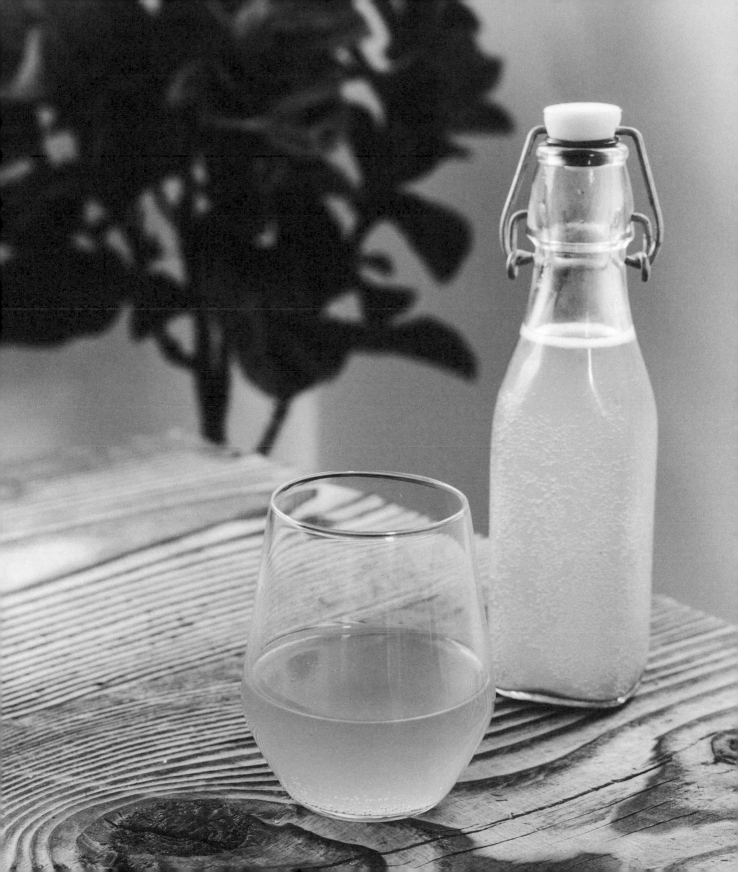

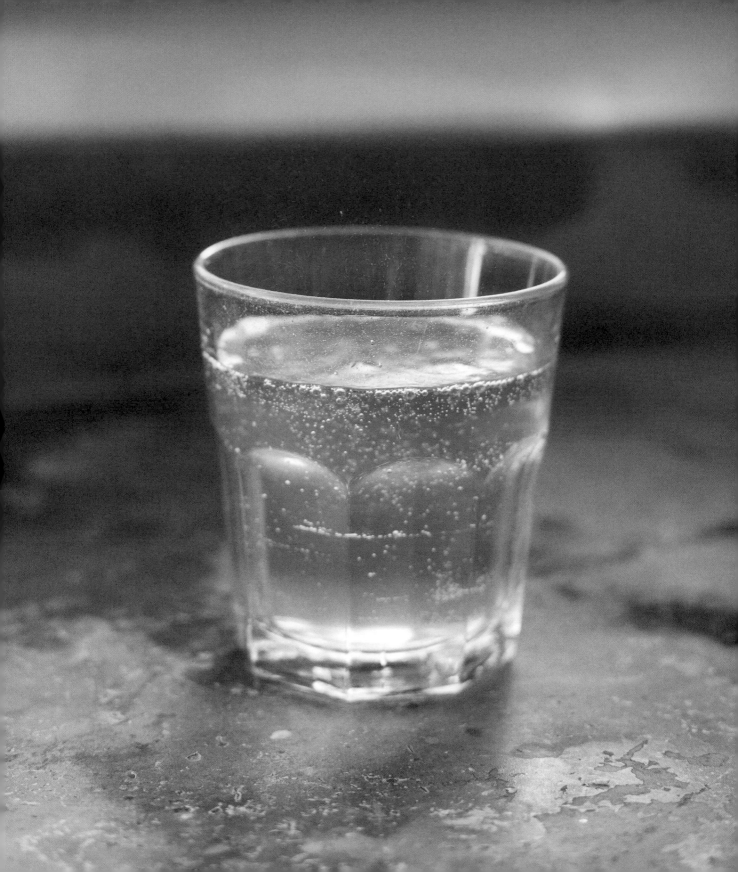

WATER KEFIR

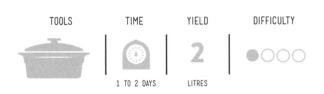

TOOLS | TIME | YIELD | DIFFICULTY
1 TO 2 DAYS | 2 LITRES | ●○○○

110 g granulated sugar
   (do not use honey or agave
   here)
2 litres filtered water, at room
   temperature
4 tablespoons water-kefir
   grains*

You will also need:
2 x 1-litre glass jars
Muslin
Rubber bands

1 Place 55 g of the sugar in each of the glass jars and add a little bit of warm water to dissolve.

2 Divide the rest of the water between the jars, making sure it is at room temperature (if it is too warm it will kill the grains).

3 Add the grains, cover each jar with a muslin and secure with a rubber band.

4 Place on the counter for 24 to 48 hours to ferment—you should see some bubbles and it will smell slightly sour.

5 Strain out the kefir grains, bottle the liquid, and store in the refrigerator to stop the fermentation. Your kefir is ready to drink as-is or bottle ferment, and you can now use the grains to start another batch.

Bottle Fermenting: To make the kefir carbonated, put the strained water kefir back in the jars with 30 to 60 ml of fruit juice in the bottom. Place an airtight lid on and let bottle-ferment for a couple of days on the countertop, remembering to 'burp' or open the lids once a day to let the gasses escape. When they are finished, put into the refrigerator and enjoy!

*Note: You can find starter cultures (also called 'grains') at some natural groceries and online—or you may have a friend who has a batch that has multiplied. The grains resemble a wobbly cottage cheese and may increase in numbers with subsequent batches. If you buy online, sometimes the cultures come dehydrated, so you will need to follow the rehydrating instructions before following this recipe.

Storage: Water kefir keeps for a month in the refrigerator.

RENDERED ANIMAL FAT

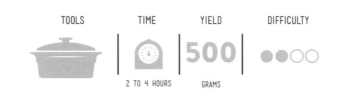

TOOLS	TIME	YIELD	DIFFICULTY
	2 TO 4 HOURS	500 GRAMS	●●○○

500 g cold animal fat (lard, tallow, duck fat or suet work well), cold

60 ml water

1 Cut the fat into small pieces—ideally smaller than 2.5 cm. Place them in a large cast-iron pot or a slow-cooker with the water and turn the heat to the lowest setting.

2 Let the fat cook on low for an hour or so, stirring every so often.

3 Once there is a considerable amount of fat melted (maybe a third to a half of the solid fat), strain most of it through a fine sieve into another pot, leaving about 60 ml in with the solid fat and set aside. Place the remaining unrendered fat back on the stove. Continue doing this until there is only a small amount of unrendered fat in the pot.

4 Once all of the fat is in the second pot and warm enough to be liquefied but not still hot, transfer into a glass jar for storage.

Note: You can take the solids (the cracklings) left in the pot after the rendering process and bake them for 20 minutes at 200°C. They make a great crunchy snack or salad topping!

Sourcing Note: Make sure to use fat from healthy animals—those that have been raised on free-range farms and fed an appropriate diet.

Storage: Keeps for a few months in the refrigerator. Also freezes well.

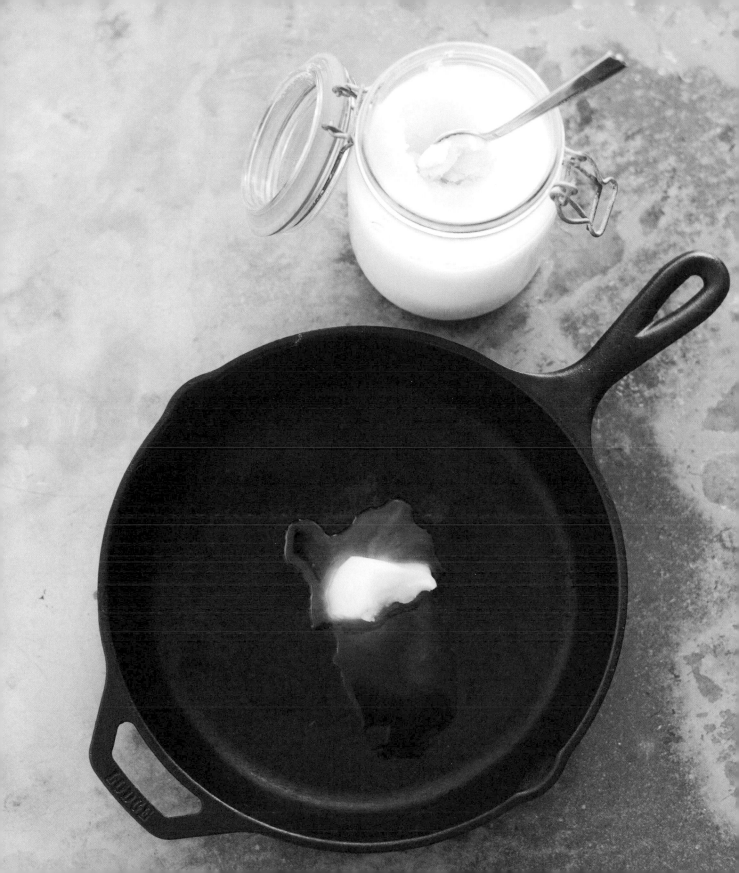

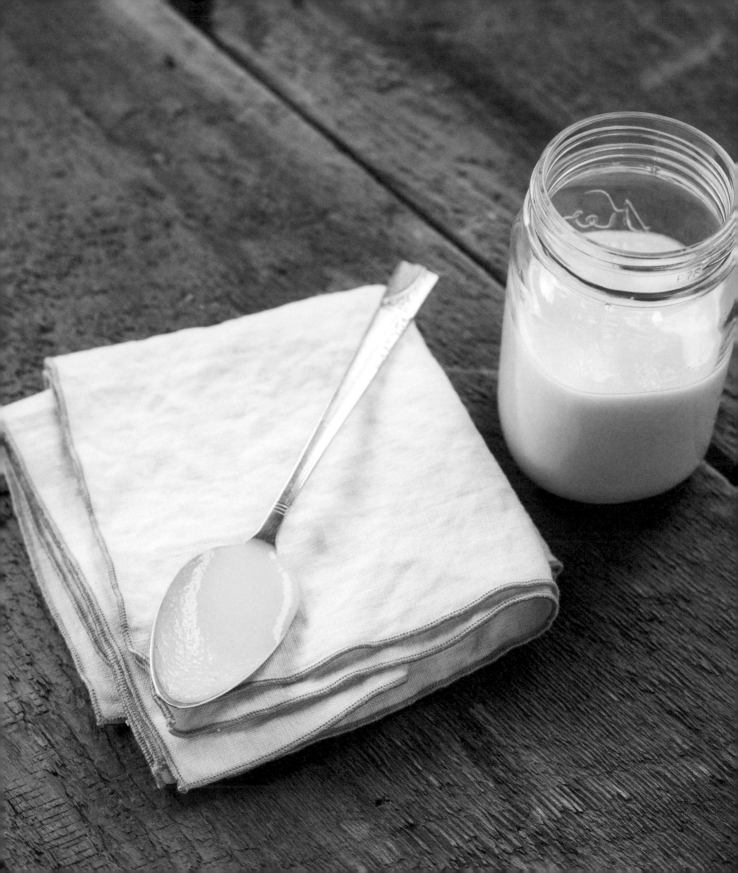

COCONUT CONCENTRATE

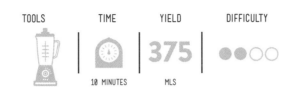

TOOLS	TIME	YIELD	DIFFICULTY
	10 MINUTES	375 MLS	●●○○

260 g dried, fine shredded
   coconut (unsweetened)
1 tablespoon coconut oil
Sea salt to taste

You will also need:
High-powered blender
or food processor

1 Place the coconut flakes, coconut oil and salt in the blender.

2 Process on high speed, while pushing down with a tamper (you may have to stop and do this manually if you are using a food processor). Process for about a minute at a time, taking breaks so as to not overheat the motor. After about 5 to 10 minutes, you should be left with a thick, creamy paste.

3 Pour into a glass jar.

Storage: Keeps well at room temperature for a few months.

CREAMY COCONUT MILK

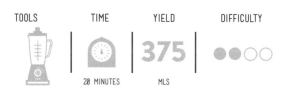

TOOLS | TIME | YIELD | DIFFICULTY
20 MINUTES | 375 MLS | ●●○○

65 g fine shredded coconut
(unsweetened)
500 ml boiling filtered water
Sea salt, to taste

You will also need:
Blender
Muslin

1 Place the shredded coconut and boiling water in your blender and blend on high speed for a few minutes, taking breaks for the motor if needed.

2 Let cool for at least 15 minutes—until it can be safely handled. Taste and season, if needed, then strain through a fine muslin into a glass jar.

Note: Keeps for a few days stored in the refrigerator. The cream will separate from the liquid, so shake or heat gently before using.

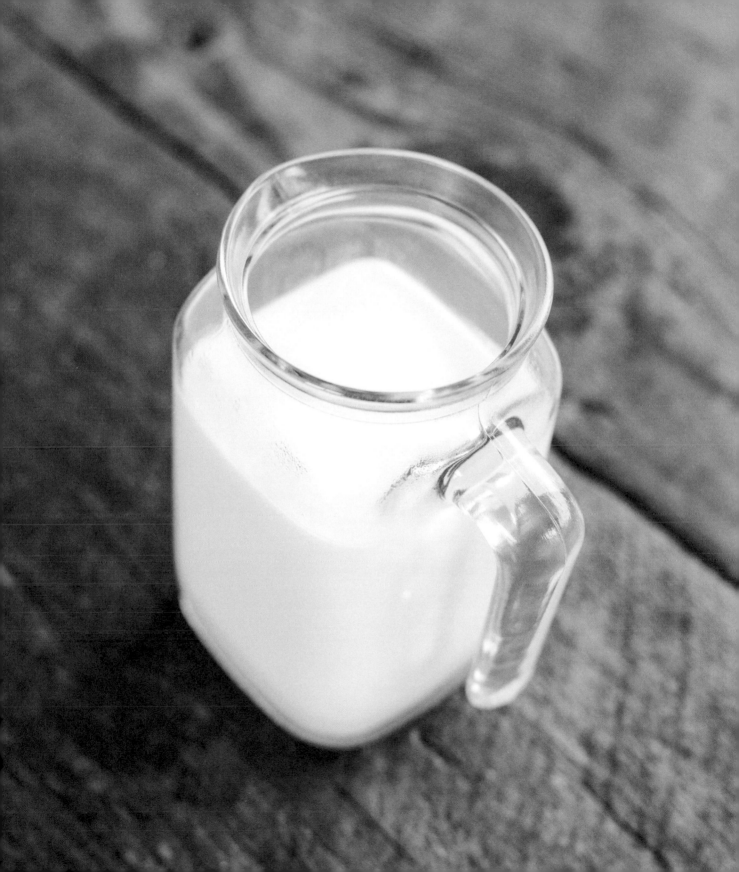

RECOMMENDED TOOLS

· Heavy-bottomed casserole – Having a versatile, heavy-bottomed casserole that can go from the stovetop to the oven and has a tight-fitting lid is very handy.

· Roasting tin and baking trays – You will need at least one sturdy baking tray and one deep roasting tin.

· Cast-iron frying pan – It's great to have a seasoned cast-iron frying pan on hand for browning meats and sautéing on the stovetop. Another plus is that it can go in the oven and double as a small roasting pan.

· Chef's knife – You need at least one good, sharp knife for slicing meat and chopping vegetables. For all of the cooking you are going to be doing on the protocol, it is worth it to have a nice, sharp knife!

· Mixing bowls – You want at least two sizeable mixing bowls (stainless steel is lightweight and durable) for prepping food and tossing salads.

· Spoons and utensils – It's good to have a variety of utensils for cooking. Make sure you have a pair of tongs, a couple of large wooden stirring spoons, a spatula and a whisk.

· Cutting board – If you are sharing a house with others who may be eating food not included on the protocol, you may want to invest in a separate cutting board. I like wooden boards that have feet so they don't warp with constant washing.

· High-powered blender – This appliance is kind of a splurge, but really makes food prep a lot easier. In addition to making smoothies and sauces like a regular blender, the high-powered variety can handle things like coconut butter, emulsions, sorbet and thick sauces.

· Glass storage containers – Portion-size glass storage containers are incredibly useful for storing leftovers in the refrigerator. Be sure to get ones with BPA-free lids.

· Meat thermometer – It's a really good idea to have a decent meat thermometer, especially if you plan on cooking a lot of poultry.

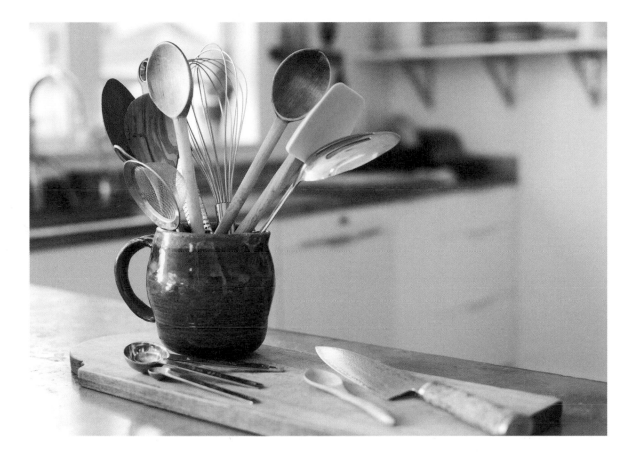

• **Little tools** – Having some assorted little tools makes some tasks easier—I like having a spiralizer, mandoline, microplane zester and vegetable peeler. You should also have a set of measuring cups and spoons.

• **Extras** – Some unnecessary, slightly fancy tools would be a pressure cooker to make bone broth more quickly, a food processor (especially if you don't have a high-powered blender), and a juicer. You definitely don't need these tools to try the protocol, but they do make some tasks easier.

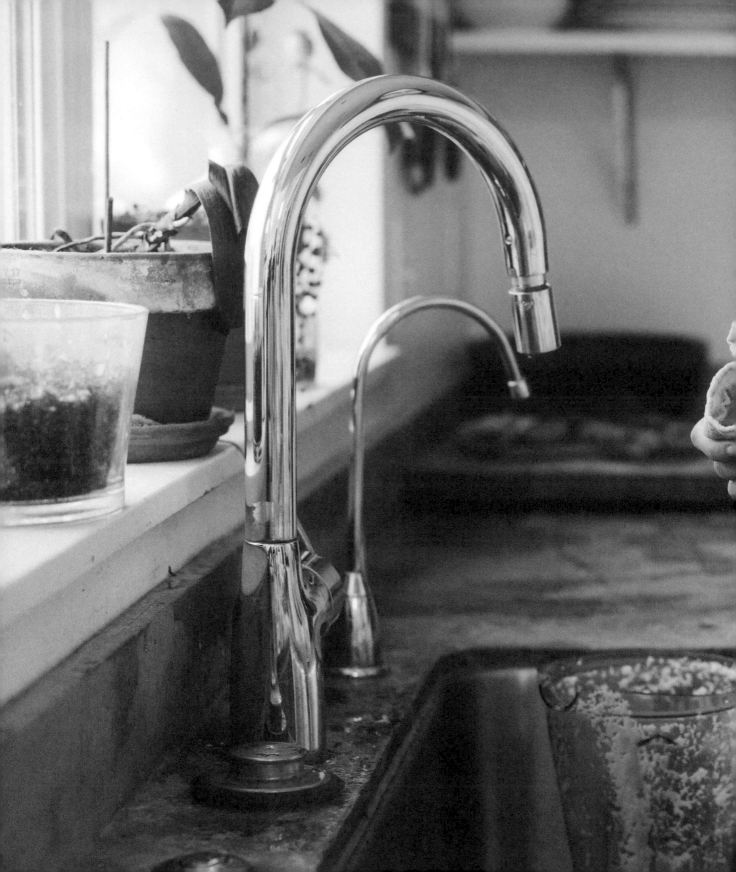

TIPS + TRICKS

HOW TO USE THIS BOOK

All the recipes in this book are suitable for the Autoimmune Protocol (known in Sarah Ballantyne's work as *The Paleo Approach*). Although most people end up expanding the list of foods they can tolerate, I wanted to create a resource for those at the beginning of the process. If you don't want to jump in right away and instead are interested in a slower transition, I encourage you to try some recipes to get your feet wet—I think you'll be surprised at how easy and palatable they are!

It is my hope that you use the meal plans as a template, making modifications and substitutions as you go to reflect your preferences and the availability of ingredients in your area. I know there are many people with digestive issues who would need to eliminate certain vegetables, and in that case, I want you to get comfortable making additions and substitutions. For instance, if you don't tolerate sweet potato, substitute butternut squash. If you are avoiding onions or garlic, leave them out and substitute ginger. If you prefer Swiss chard over kale, go for it! My goal is to give you the tools to cook simple, flavourful meals that can easily be customised to your preferences or the season.

A Note On Sugar

Although it is well known that sugar can cause autoimmune flares, this is not a completely sugar-free cookbook. I have included some fruit for flavouring within the context of a balanced meal—one with adequate protein and fat. I have also included a small dessert section; most of those recipes are fruit-sweetened, but there are a couple with maple syrup or honey. I don't advise including excessive fruit or sugar (even from natural sources like maple syrup or honey) while on the protocol, but I wanted to include those recipes for a special occasion or a treat if needed. I guess this is a warning to not go crazy in this department—it will hinder your progress!

A Note On Cooking Fat

Instead of specifying which fat to use in the recipes, I call for 'solid cooking fat'. This can be any fat of your choosing, as long as it is saturated and solid at room temperature: coconut oil, lard, tallow, duck fat, among others. Sometimes I have specified coconut oil when the recipe requires a more neutral flavour, but don't be afraid to substitute if you would like to use something else. I have included a recipe for rendering your own fat on page 42.

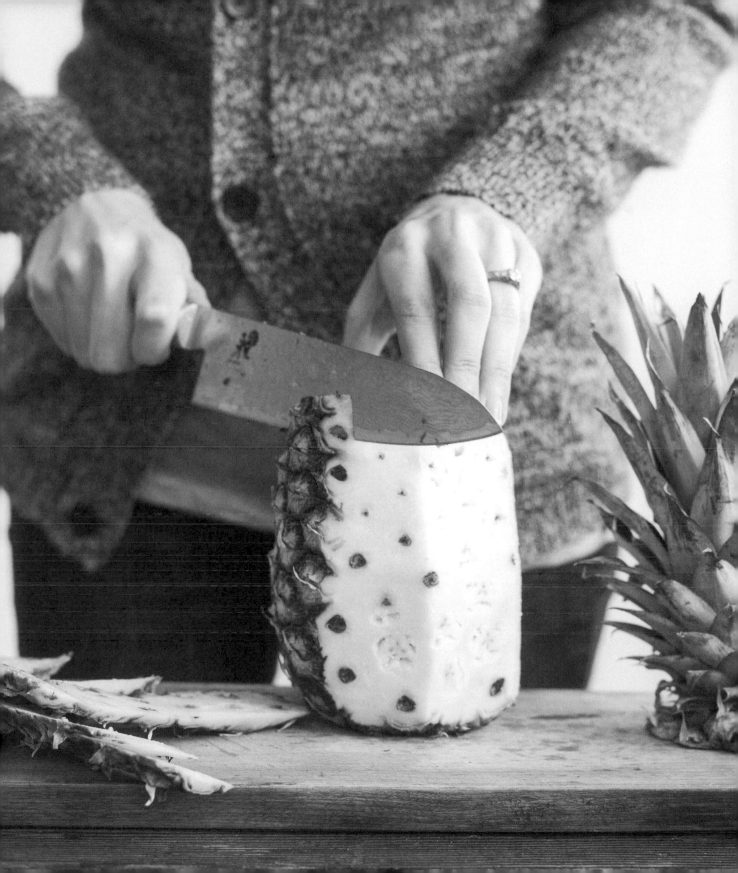

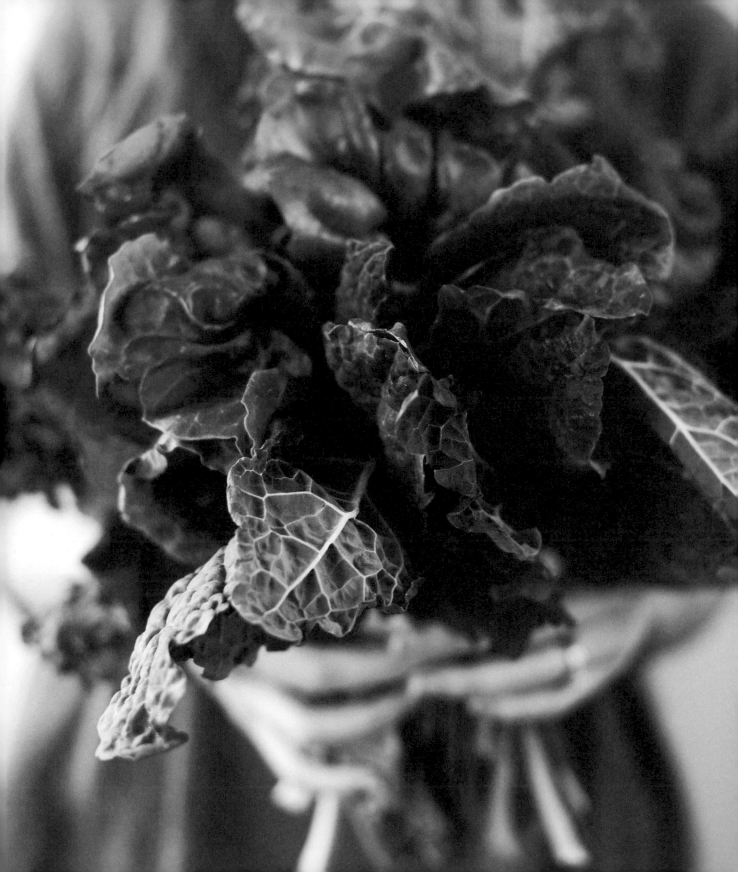

A NOTE ON FOOD QUALITY

The Autoimmune Protocol removes gut irritants and common potential allergens, replacing them with whole, nourishing foods and thereby removing all of the commercial processed foods that are so prevalent in our modern society. Simply avoiding certain foods and eating others is not the entire plan, however; food quality plays a critical role when you are on a mission to heal and nourish your body. It is well known that the nutritional value of food can vary greatly, depending on how it was grown or raised—and when our goal is to seek out those nutrients that enable our bodies to heal, the search to find high-quality food becomes very important.

Before you run off to your local health-food store and pay lots of money for products that are raised organically/free-range/grass-fed, you may want to do some research into what is available locally and seasonally to cut down on costs (often times these products also end up being more healthy for us *and* the planet!). If you're on a budget and can't afford the highest quality of everything, prioritise and go from there. Don't assume that because you can't afford organic-market prices for high-quality food it is out of your budget. Buying in bulk, shopping seasonally, volunteering at a farmers' market, shopping online, starting a garden and frequenting a few different stores are all smart strategies that will cut costs while keeping food quality high.

SHOPPING GUIDE

Meat: It is very important to buy hormone-free meat, at the very least. Of course organic, grass-fed, and free-range are preferable, but it is unrealistic to expect that everyone has the access or budget to afford it. If you can't afford grass-fed or free-range all the time, try buying the tougher, fattier cuts of meat (which are usually cheaper anyway) grass-fed and the leaner cuts at least hormone-free. Also, buying in bulk directly from a farmer saves a tonne over paying premium prices at the store—check out the resources on page 303 to find a farm near you. A deep freezer is great for storing a bulk meat order, as well as a place to freeze extra meat you might find on sale at the store or farmers' market. In the case of fish, always be sure to buy wild-caught varieties—not farmed. Tinned fish should be packed in BPA-free tins and free of fillers and other ingredients.

Fats/Oils: Olive and avocado oils are the only unsaturated oils (liquid at room temperature) that I recommend on the Autoimmune Protocol. Do not buy any nut or seed oils (sesame, walnut, canola). Be sure to buy brands that are cold-pressed and come in opaque bottles. Only use liquid oils for cold applications, like salad dressings or to drizzle on raw vegetables. For cooking, always use some form of solid fat, either of tropical or animal origin. Coconut oil is a great staple for cooking and one I use often in my kitchen. Animal fats are also a good choice, as long as they come from a good source (free-range animals), as toxins are often stored in the fat. If you are willing to render your own fat (page 42), chunks of lard, tallow and sometimes duck fat can be purchased from many farmers quite inexpensively.

Produce: If you cannot get all organic produce, use the reference lists of the most toxic non-organic produce to guide your purchases. Buying locally and in season is always preferable and usually the most cost effective. If you have a cool place to store them, root vegetables like squashes, sweet potatoes and onions can be purchased in bulk. Farmers' markets or local co-operative farm shops are always the best source for produce if you can manage to find one in your area, followed by health-food stores. Don't assume that you have to travel great distances to find organic produce these days, as most conventional supermarkets have increasingly more varieties and better prices on organic goods.

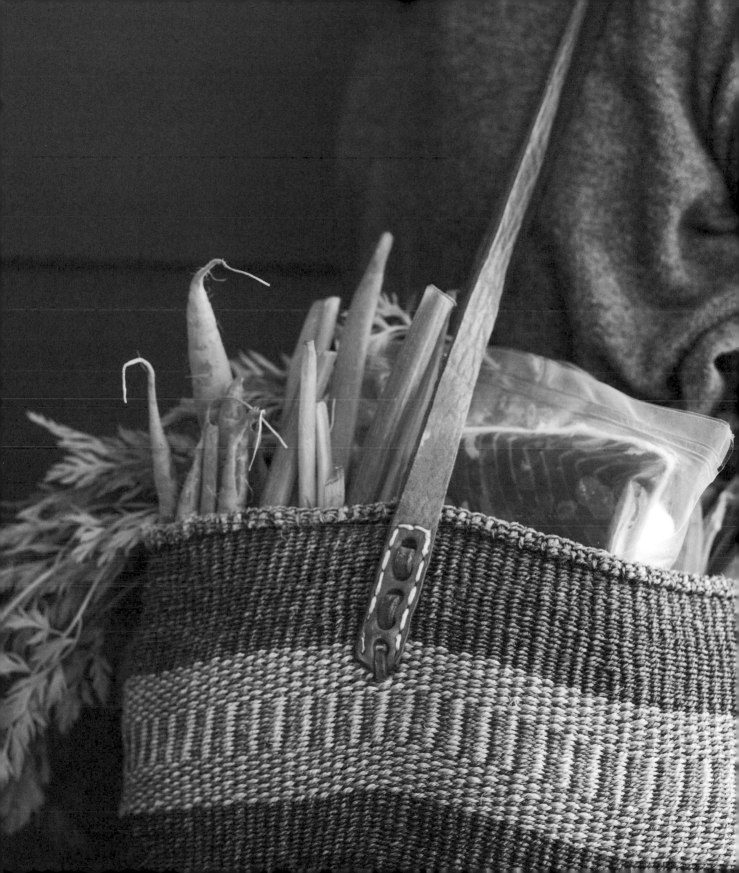

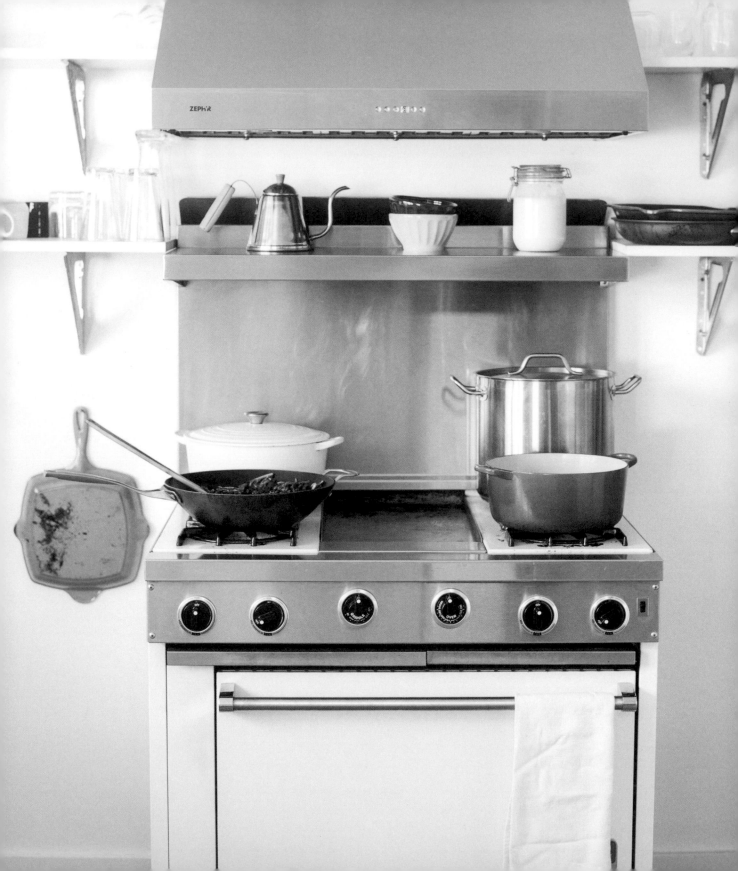

A NOTE ON BATCH COOKING

One of the biggest ways to make the Autoimmune Protocol go more smoothly is to incorporate weekly batch cooking into your routine, especially if you are crunched for time during the work week. Because the Autoimmune Protocol excludes all processed foods, everything must be cooked from scratch. This can be extremely problematic for someone who works full time, cares for children or is very ill. On the next page, I have compiled some ideas to get you started on planning a batch-cooking routine and help you make sure that you always have nutrient-dense meal components ready to go.

BATCH-COOKING IDEAS

• **Bone Broth** – Make this once a week (page 34) and store in glass jars for use in soups, stews and for drinking with breakfast instead of coffee. If you really want to get ahead, make two batches at the same time and freeze one of them.

• **Meat Patties** – Homemade meat patties are the best security blanket on the Autoimmune Protocol. Make a batch or two once a week and freeze the patties between slices of waxed paper. You can make a few different kinds: Three-Herb Beef (page 262), Garlic-Sage Chicken (page 211) or Rosemary-Mint Lamb (page 269)—then you always have a quick, clean source of protein and some variety to choose from. Homemade meat patties are the fastest protein for breakfast—just reheat them gently in a frying pan. You can also use them for a quick meal or a snack if you run short of other options.

• **Soups/Stews** – When making a soup or stew, it's a great idea to double the recipe and freeze half of it in portion-size containers. Then you can pull one out to thaw overnight for a lunch at work or a quick meal.

• **Meat** – It's great to get in the habit of cooking a big batch of meat to add to meals over the following days. For instance, you can make the Herbed Roast Chicken (page 227), pull off all of the meat, and then use the carcass to make bone broth. Then you can reserve the meat to add to salads, lettuce cups and stir-fries. Making a big batch of Shredded Roast Beef (page 261) or Shredded Chicken Breast (page 212) is also great for this. Save recipes that are time consuming for your batch-cooking day, and then the days following you can just use the meat to assemble meals with some quickly cooked vegetables.

• **Staples** – Make staples like Creamy Coconut Milk (page 46), Coconut Concentrate (page 45), Garlic 'Mayo' (page 127), Coconut-Basil Pesto (page 124), Nomato Sauce (page 135) and other dressings and sauces that keep well on your batch-cooking day. Then you'll have an assortment of components to draw on for recipes and meals.

THOUGHTS ON BREAKFAST

When people think of a breakfast, even a so-called 'healthy' one, it's hard not to conjure up images of grains and eggs. The Autoimmune Protocol does not lend itself well to traditional breakfast-type foods, with the possible exceptions of bacon and sausage (and even sausages usually contain nightshade spices). Because of this, I have not included a breakfast category in the cookbook. This is perhaps one of the most difficult concepts for people to get once they decide to start eating this way. The only thing that makes breakfast different from lunch or dinner on this plan is that it is generally a meal that needs to be prepared more quickly than usual. For this reason, it's even more ideal to have pre-prepared meals or components on hand.

I think it is important to make breakfast the most hearty, satisfying meal of the day. I know this is hard for those who are not hungry in the morning, or those who are used to drinking a cup of coffee and running out the door. If you don't like eating breakfast, start increasing the quality and quantity of your morning meal gradually, and you might find that your morning hunger improves. Be sure to include a few ounces of protein and some fat at breakfast, as this is very important to keep your blood sugar stable and keep you satiated for the rest of the day. Remember: healing bodies need lots of quality fuel, and breakfast is a perfect time to get these nutrients in.

My favorite breakfasts are those that combine foods I have prepared ahead of time, like sausage patties or other protein, leftover vegetables or fresh cooked greens, some fermented vegetables, a mug of bone broth and maybe a slice of fruit or rasher of bacon to round out the plate. All of these items are readily available in my kitchen, and I can easily piece together a nourishing and nutrient-dense meal in a matter of minutes. On the next page I've given you some examples of foods to have available to create a satisfying and healing breakfast.

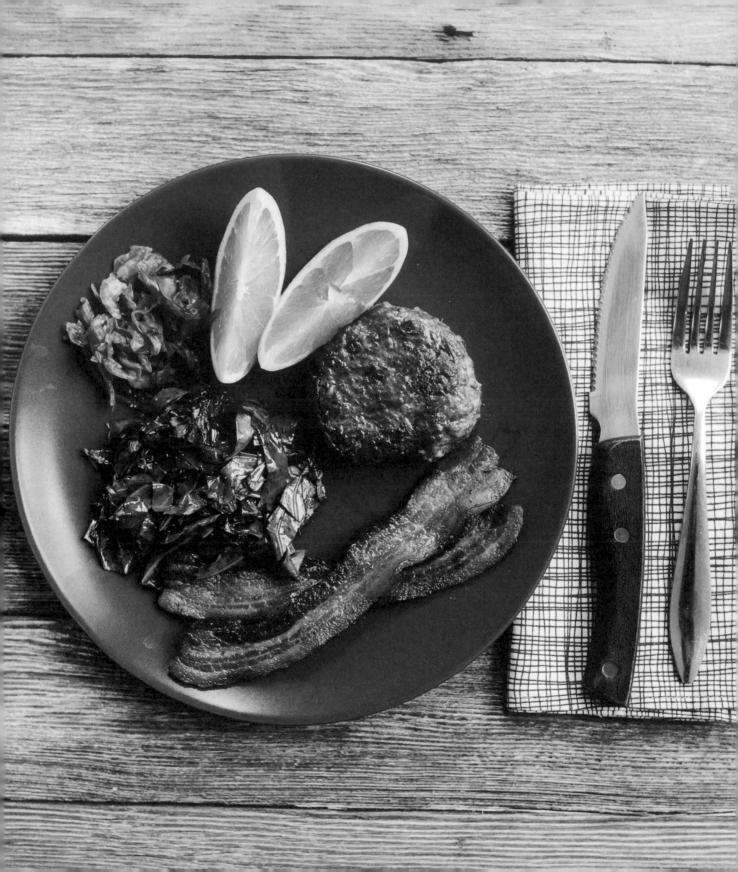

BREAKFAST IDEAS

- **Meat Patties** - If you have at least two different kinds in your freezer, you can avoid having the same thing for breakfast every morning. Just grab one out of the freezer and reheat it in a frying pan. Try the Three-Herb Breakfast Patties (page 262), Garlic-Sage Chicken Patties (page 211) or Rosemary-Mint Lamb Patties (page 269).

- **Bone Broth** - Breakfast is a great time to enjoy a mug of broth! It can replace your morning coffee or tea, or you can add some leftover vegetables and meat to create a quick soup. My recipe is on page 34.

- **Fermented Vegetables** - Sauerkraut (page 37) or other fermented vegetables can be stored in your fridge and just scooped out onto your plate to add to breakfast.

- **Leftover Vegetables** - If you have any leftover veggies from your dinner the day before, you can throw them into the frying pan to heat up with the meat patties. You can also batch-cook a big vegetable hash every week to quickly reheat for breakfasts.

- **Raw Fruit or Vegetables** - You can eat a piece of fruit or some raw vegetables with your breakfast, but I would not choose this in lieu of quality protein or fat.

- **Tinned Fish** - If you run out of patties or are in a rush, a BPA-free tin of fish (salmon or sardines are nice) mashed up with some raw veggies can be a quick solution.

- **Bacon** - Always a nice addition to breakfast. Be sure to purchase a free-range, sugar-free variety.

- **Leftover Meals** - Forget your prior perception of breakfast. If you have a leftover portion of stew or other hearty meal with a serving of protein, eat it for breakfast!

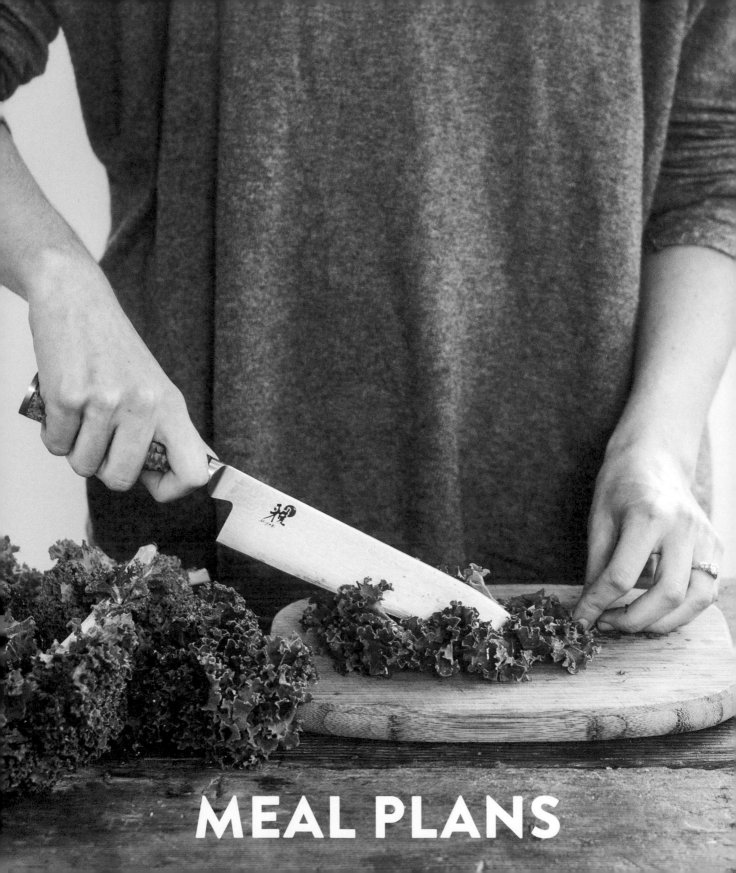

MEAL PLANS

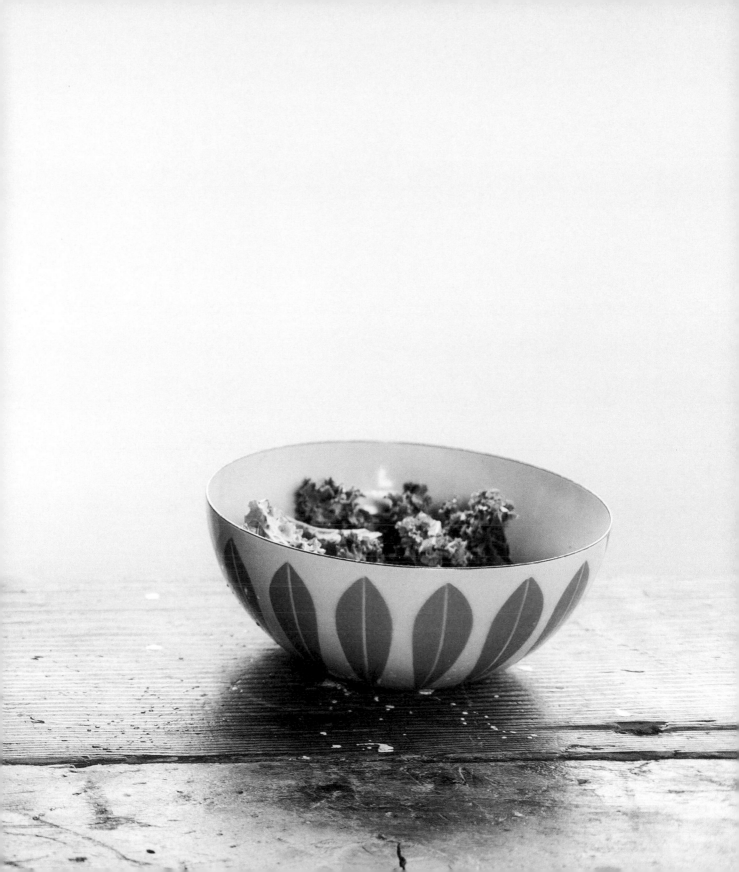

ABOUT THE MEAL PLANS

On the following pages I have included two meal plans that each cover a month's worth of meals, including shopping lists for the corresponding recipes. For these meal plans I've selected recipes that are easy to make, palatable to a wide variety of preferences, and keep well enough to be eaten as leftovers throughout the week. My goal in organising information this way is to give those who may be new to this style of eating a concrete plan so that they can set themselves up to be successful in their transition. By the end of the month, you should be very comfortable working with a wide range of ingredients and ready to branch out and make your own weekly meal plans. Because most people are busy or work a traditional schedule, I have scheduled the bulk of the cooking to happen on the weekends and at dinnertime. All lunches on the plan are leftovers that may be taken to work or prepared quickly on the go.

The Complete Four-Week Meal Plan is what I would recommend for those coming to the Autoimmune Protocol for the first time, especially if they are transitioning from a standard Western diet. This is a very plentiful, nourishing diet, and I have erred on the side of caution when planning food portions—there should be more food rather than not enough. Changing to a very restrictive diet can be challenging if there is not enough food available, and I have allowed so that a person following this plan will always have some extra food available in case they get hungry between meals.

The Alternate Four-Week Meal Plan is for those who don't want to eat meat at every meal, for either personal preference or because of budget concerns. Although I recommend having at least a small serving of meat at every meal, I wanted to make a plan for those who could only afford a certain amount of high-quality meat or were put off by the thought of eating so much of it. This plan is similar to the complete plan except that there is no meat at lunchtime.

A FEW NOTES BEFORE YOU START

• The meal plans account for one person for four weeks. As I said previously, the plans both account for generous servings of food, in an effort to avoid a situation where a person is hungry but doesn't have anything available to eat. If you find that you have excess food prepared, drop some of the vegetable side dishes and eat leftovers instead.

• Meals that need to be cooked from scratch are denoted in colour and correspond to page numbers for the recipes in the book. You can easily glance at the week and see which meals you will need to cook from scratch. All of the meals in black have already been prepped or cooked previously and should only take a quick reheat or assembly.

• I have accounted for 115 g to 175 g of meat per meal in the shopping lists. If you want to eat more or less, adjust your shopping list and recipes accordingly.

• There are twice-weekly shopping lists that take into consideration how long the meat will last in the refrigerator, but you have the option of buying all the meat for a week and then freezing some portions for later. Generally meat takes 24 to 48 hours to thaw in the refrigerator, so plan accordingly; you want to have your meat ready to go when you're ready to cook.

• There is a list of pantry items to be stocked while on the meal plan on each shopping list. These are items that store well and are commonly used—like onions, vinegar and sea salt. It is assumed that as you run out of them, you will stock up.

• For breakfasts, I have only included the meat component. I suggest completing the meal with leftover vegetables, fermented vegetables, bone broth, or items like avocados, bacon or fruit. Getting in the hang of assembling a great breakfast takes some planning, but after a few days you will find a combination and amount that suits you and fuels your day.

COMPLETE 4-WEEK MEAL PLAN

WEEK 1

	BREAKFAST	LUNCH	DINNER
SUNDAY	Three-Herb Beef Patties (page 262) (also make Garlic-Sage Chicken Patties page 211)	Citrus-Ginger Marinated Salmon (page 237) Cauliflower 'Fried Rice' (page 200)	Classic Chicken Soup (page 165)*
MONDAY	Three-Herb Beef Patties	Classic Chicken Soup	Citrus-Ginger Marinated Salmon Cauliflower 'Fried Rice'
TUESDAY	Garlic-Sage Chicken Patties	Citrus-Ginger Marinated Salmon Cauliflower 'Fried Rice'	Garlic Beef and Broccoli (page 270)*** Radish and Jicama Tabbouli (page 142)
WEDNESDAY	Mediterranean Salmon Salad (page 153)	Classic Chicken Soup	Shredded Chicken Breast (page 212) Curried Chicken Salad (page 224) Emerald Kale Salad (page 138)
THURSDAY	Mediterranean Salmon Salad	Garlic Beef and Broccoli Radish and Jicama Tabbouli	Curried Chicken Salad Emerald Kale Salad
FRIDAY	Three-Herb Beef Patties	Curried Chicken Salad Emerald Kale Salad	Mediterranean Salmon (page 242) Rosemary Grilled Asparagus (page 195) Sautéed Market Greens (page 183)
SATURDAY	Three-Herb Beef Patties	Mediterranean Salmon Rosemary Grilled Asparagus Sautéed Market Greens	Beef-Butternut Stew with Pear and Thyme (page 161)**

*Freeze two servings **Freeze one serving ***Halve recipe

WEEK 2

	BREAKFAST	LUNCH	DINNER
SUNDAY	Garlic-Sage Chicken Patties	Mediterranean Salmon Rosemary Grilled Asparagus Sautéed Market Greens	Beef-Butternut Stew with Pear and Thyme Shredded Roast Beef (page 261) (save for later in week)**
MONDAY	Mediterranean Salmon Salad (page 153)	Beef-Butternut Stew with Pear and Thyme	Shredded Chicken Breast (page 212) Chicken Stir-Fry (page 231) Curried Cauliflower (page 187)
TUESDAY	Mediterranean Salmon Salad	Chicken Stir-Fry Curried Cauliflower	Coconut Amino–Marinated Salmon (page 237) Cabbage Slaw with Olive-Avocado Dressing (page 145)
WEDNESDAY	Garlic-Sage Chicken Patties	Coconut Amino–Marinated Salmon Cabbage Slaw with Olive-Avocado Dressing	Rosemary Shredded Beef (page 278) Emerald Kale Salad (page 138)
THURSDAY	Garlic-Sage Chicken Patties	Coconut Amino–Marinated Salmon Cabbage Slaw with Olive-Avocado Dressing	Rosemary Shredded Beef Emerald Kale Salad
FRIDAY	Garlic-Sage Chicken Patties	Rosemary Shredded Beef Emerald Kale Salad	Asian Marinated Grilled Chicken (page 219) Carrot-Ginger Soup (page 162)*
SATURDAY	Three-Herb Beef Patties (page 262) (also make Garlic-Sage Chicken Patties page 211)	Asian Marinated Grilled Chicken Carrot-Ginger Soup	Citrus-Ginger Marinated Salmon (page 237) Market Salad (page 149)

*Freeze one serving **Halve recipe

COMPLETE 4-WEEK MEAL PLAN

WEEK 3

	BREAKFAST	LUNCH	DINNER
SUNDAY	Garlic-Sage Chicken Patties	Citrus-Ginger Marinated Salmon Market Salad	Cinnamon-Sage Dry-Rub Steak (page 265)** Brussels Sprouts with Crispy Bacon (page 191)
MONDAY	Three-Herb Beef Patties	Cinnamon-Sage Dry-Rub Steak Brussels Sprouts with Crispy Bacon	Lemon-Garlic Marinated Chicken (page 219) Market Salad
TUESDAY	Three-Herb Beef Patties	Lemon-Garlic Marinated Chicken Brussels Sprouts with Crispy Bacon	Classic Tuna Salad (page 232) Mashed Sweet Potatoes (page 192)*
WEDNESDAY	Mediterranean Salmon Salad (page 153)	Classic Tuna Salad Mashed Sweet Potatoes	Classic Chicken Soup (frozen; thawed day prior)
THURSDAY	Mediterranean Salmon Salad	Classic Chicken Soup (frozen; thawed two days prior)	Shredded Chicken Breast (page 212) Chicken and Pesto Sauté (page 216) Rainbow Roasted Root Vegetables (page 188)
FRIDAY	Three-Herb Beef Patties	Classic Tuna Salad Mashed Sweet Potatoes	Chicken and Pesto Sauté Rainbow Roasted Root Vegetables
SATURDAY	Garlic-Sage Chicken Patties	Sole Fillet with Tarragon-Caper Sauce (page 245) Puréed Parsnips (page 196)	Herbed Dry-Rub Steak (page 265)** Sautéed Market Greens (page 183) Rainbow Roasted Root Vegetables

*Thaw two servings of soup **Halve recipe

WEEK 4

	BREAKFAST	LUNCH	DINNER
SUNDAY	Garlic-Sage Chicken Patties	Sole Fillet with Tarragon-Caper Sauce Sautéed Market Greens Puréed Parsnips	Shredded Roast Beef (page 261) Lettuce Cups Mango Salsa (page 131)
MONDAY	Garlic-Sage Chicken Patties	Shredded Roast Beef Lettuce Boats Mango Salsa	Sole Fillet with Tarragon-Caper Sauce Sautéed Market Greens Puréed Parsnips
TUESDAY	Mediterranean Salmon Salad (page 153)	Shredded Roast Beef Lettuce Cups Mango Salsa	Sage-Braised Chicken Legs (page 228)** Puréed Parsnips (page 196)
WEDNESDAY	Mediterranean Salmon Salad	Sage-Braised Chicken Legs Puréed Parsnips	'Spaghetti' and Meatballs (page 282)** Cinnamon-Scented Butternut Squash (page 184)
THURSDAY	Three-Herb Beef Patties	'Spaghetti' and Meatballs Cinnamon-Scented Butternut Squash	Salmon Salad with Olives and Cucumber (page 238) Cucumber-Mint Salad (page 141)*
FRIDAY	Garlic-Sage Chicken Patties	Salmon Salad with Olives and Cucumber Cucumber-Mint Salad	Beef-Butternut Stew with Pear and Thyme (frozen; thawed day prior) Cinnamon-Scented Butternut Squash*
SATURDAY	Garlic-Sage Chicken Patties	Salmon Salad with Olives and Cucumber Emerald Kale Salad (page 138)	Herbed Dry-Rub Steak (page 265)*** Carrot-Ginger Soup (frozen; thawed day prior) Emerald Kale Salad

*Thaw one serving of soup **Halve recipe ***Quarter recipe

COMPLETE 4-WEEK MEAL PLANNER

	WEEK 1	WEEK 2
PANTRY ITEMS	**SATURDAY**	**SATURDAY**

<table>
<tr><td>

PANTRY ITEMS

solid cooking fat of your
   choice (lard, tallow, duck
   fat, etc.)
coconut oil
extra-virgin olive oil
coconut concentrate
ground ginger
ground turmeric
dried sage
ground cinnamon
bay leaves
sea salt
coconut flour
kalamata olives
capers
apple cider vinegar
coconut aminos
shredded coconut flakes

</td><td>

900 g grass-fed ground beef
900 g chicken thigh, ground
1 x 1.8–2.25 kg free-range chicken
680 g wild-caught salmon
450 g grass-fed sirloin steak
900 g carrots
1 bunch celery
1 bunch radishes
225 g jicama
1 courgette (zucchini)
2 cucumbers
1 bunch broccolini
1 head cauliflower
90 g mushrooms
2 oranges
fresh chives
fresh mint
fresh flat-leaf parsley (large bunch)
fresh rosemary
fresh sage (2 bunches)
fresh thyme

</td><td>

900 g beef brisket or stewing beef
900 g beef brisket
450 g wild-caught salmon
450 g free-range chicken breast
1 large butternut squash
900 g carrots
450 g broccoli
270 g mushrooms
1 head cauliflower
1 small head savoy cabbage
1–2 avocados
2 firm pears
fresh flat-leaf parsley
fresh thyme

</td></tr>
</table>

KEEP IN STOCK	**WEDNESDAY**	**WEDNESDAY**

<table>
<tr><td>

KEEP IN STOCK

onions
red onions
fresh garlic
fresh ginger
lemons
BPA-free tinned salmon
BPA-free tinned tuna

HAVE READY

fermented vegetables
   (page 37)
bone broth (page 34)
garlic 'mayo' (page 127)

</td><td>

450 g wild-caught salmon
450 g free-range chicken breast
1 small cucumber
3 bunches dark leafy greens
   (kale, chard, spring greens)
900 g asparagus
1 head lettuce
fresh flat-leaf parsley
fresh rosemary
45 g raisins

</td><td>

450 g free-range chicken breast
2 large sweet potatoes
900 g carrots
2 courgettes (zucchini)
1 bunch kale
1 small cucumber
1 orange
fresh chives
fresh rosemary

</td></tr>
</table>

SHOPPING LIST

WEEK 3	WEEK 4
SATURDAY	**SATURDAY**

900 g grass-fed beef mince
900 g chicken thigh, minced
450 g wild-caught salmon
450 g free-range chicken breast
450 g grass-fed steak
6 rashers sugar-free bacon
900 g sweet potatoes
680 g brussels sprouts
45 g mushrooms
1 head lettuce
1 head romaine lettuce
3 carrots
1 bunch celery
1 beetroot
1 cucumber
1 avocado
2 oranges
fresh dill
fresh mint
fresh flat-leaf parsley
fresh rosemary
fresh sage
fresh thyme
	900 g beef brisket
	350 g grass-fed steak
	680 g free-range chicken legs
	   and thighs
	2 large bunches of dark leafy greens
	   (kale, spring greens, chard)
	680 g parsnips
	1 head romaine lettuce
	1–2 bunches spinach
	2 cucumbers
	180 g mushrooms
	1 bunch radishes
	1 avocado
	1 mango
	1 lime
	fresh coriander (large bunch)
	fresh flat-leaf parsley
	fresh sage (2 bunches)

WEDNESDAY	**WEDNESDAY**
450 g free-range chicken breast 450 g sole, flounder or John Dory fillets 680 g parsnips 450 g broccoli or broccolini 5 carrots 3 beetroots 3 parsnips 1 swede fresh basil (2 bunches) fresh tarragon 125 ml coconut water (optional)	450 g grass-fed beef mince 175 g grass-fed steak 1.3 kg butternut squash 2 beetroots 2 carrots 4 courgettes (zucchini) 1 bunch curly-leafed kale 1 bunch mixed greens or lettuce 1 cucumber fresh basil (large bunch) fresh flat-leaf parsley fresh rosemary fresh sage fresh thyme

ALTERNATE 4-WEEK MEAL PLAN

WEEK 1

	BREAKFAST	LUNCH	DINNER
SUNDAY	Three-Herb Beef Patties (page 262) (also make Garlic-Sage Chicken Patties page 211)	Hearty Vegetable Soup (page 173)*	Citrus-Ginger Marinated Salmon (page 237) Rosemary-Roasted Carrots and Parsnips (page 203) Sautéed Market Greens (page 183)
MONDAY	Three-Herb Beef Patties	Hearty Vegetable Soup	Citrus-Ginger Marinated Salmon Rosemary-Roasted Carrots and Parsnips
TUESDAY	Garlic-Sage Chicken Patties	Hearty Vegetable Soup	Garlic Beef and Broccoli (page 270)*** Cauliflower "Fried Rice" (page 200)
WEDNESDAY	Mediterranean Salmon Salad (page 153)	Cauliflower 'Fried Rice' Sautéed Market Greens	Garlic Beef and Broccoli Mashed Sweet Potatoes (page 192)
THURSDAY	Mediterranean Salmon Salad	Cauliflower 'Fried Rice' Mashed Sweet Potatoes	Shredded Chicken Breast (page 212) Curried Chicken Salad (page 224) Emerald Kale Salad (page 138)
FRIDAY	Three-Herb Beef Patties	Emerald Kale Salad Mashed Sweet Potatoes	Curried Chicken Salad Radish and Jicama Tabbouli (page 142)
SATURDAY	Garlic-Sage Chicken Patties	Emerald Kale Salad Radish and Jicama Tabbouli	Beef-Butternut Stew with Pear and Thyme (page 161)**

*Freeze three servings of soup **Freeze two servings of soup ***Halve recipe

WEEK 2

	BREAKFAST	LUNCH	DINNER
SUNDAY	Garlic-Sage Chicken Patties	Rainbow Roasted Root Vegetables (page 188) Radish and Jicama Tabbouli	Beef-Butternut Stew with Pear and Thyme Cabbage Slaw with Olive-Avocado Dressing (page 145) (prep for lunches later in week)
MONDAY	Mediterranean Salmon Salad (page 153)	Cabbage Slaw with Olive-Avocado Dressing Rainbow Roasted Root Vegetables	Beef-Butternut Stew with Pear and Thyme
TUESDAY	Mediterranean Salmon Salad	Cabbage Slaw with Olive-Avocado Dressing Rainbow Roasted Root Vegetables	'Spaghetti' and Meatballs (page 282)* Carrot-Ginger Soup (page 162)
WEDNESDAY	Garlic-Sage Chicken Patties	Cabbage Slaw with Olive-Avocado Dressing Carrot-Ginger Soup	'Spaghetti' and Meatballs Rosemary Grilled Asparagus (page 195)
THURSDAY	Three-Herb Beef Patties	Carrot-Ginger Soup Rosemary Grilled Asparagus	Mediterranean Salmon (page 242) Citrus-Spinach Salad (page 150) Sautéed Market Greens (page 183)
FRIDAY	Garlic-Sage Chicken Patties	Citrus-Spinach Salad Rosemary Grilled Asparagus	Mediterranean Salmon Sautéed Market Greens Puréed Parsnips (page 196)
SATURDAY	Three-Herb Beef Patties (page 262) (also make Garlic-Sage Chicken Patties page 211)	Citrus-Spinach Salad Sautéed Market Greens	Mediterranean Salmon Puréed Parsnips Cinnamon-Scented Butternut Squash (page 184)

*Halve recipe

ALTERNATE 4-WEEK MEAL PLAN

WEEK 3

	BREAKFAST	LUNCH	DINNER
SUNDAY	Garlic-Sage Chicken Patties	Cinnamon-Scented Butternut Squash Puréed Parsnips	Lemon-Garlic Marinated Chicken (page 219) Emerald Kale Salad (page 138)
MONDAY	Three-Herb Beef Patties	Cinnamon-Scented Butternut Squash Emerald Kale Salad	Lemon-Garlic Marinated Chicken Beetroot and Fennel Soup (page 162)*
TUESDAY	Three-Herb Beef Patties	Cinnamon-Scented Butternut Squash Emerald Kale Salad	Classic Tuna Salad (page 234) Market Salad (page 149)
WEDNESDAY	Mediterranean Salmon Salad (page 153)	Beetroot and Fennel Soup Market Salad	Classic Tuna Salad Mashed Sweet Potatoes (page 192)
THURSDAY	Mediterranean Salmon Salad	Hearty Vegetable Soup (frozen; thawed the day prior) Market Salad	Classic Tuna Salad Mashed Sweet Potatoes Roasted Mixed Vegetables (page 199)**
FRIDAY	Three-Herb Beef Patties	Mashed Sweet Potatoes Roasted Mixed Vegetables	Beef-Butternut Stew with Pear and Thyme (frozen; thawed the day prior)
SATURDAY	Garlic-Sage Chicken Patties	Curried Cauliflower (page 187) Roasted Mixed Vegetables	Beef-Butternut Stew with Pear and Thyme (frozen; thawed two days prior)

*Freeze one serving of soup **Freeze two servings of soup

WEEK 4

	BREAKFAST	LUNCH	DINNER
SUNDAY	Three-Herb Beef Patties	Curried Cauliflower Market Salad (page 149)	Sole Fillet with Tarragon-Caper Sauce (page 245) Emerald Kale Salad (page 138)* Market Salad
MONDAY	Garlic-Sage Chicken Patties	Emerald Kale Salad Hearty Vegetable Soup (frozen; thawed the day prior)	Sole Fillet with Tarragon-Caper Sauce Cucumber-Mint Salad (page 141)
TUESDAY	Mediterranean Salmon Salad (page 153)	Cucumber-Mint Salad Hearty Vegetable Soup (frozen; thawed two days prior)	Sole Fillet with Tarragon-Caper Sauce Brussels Sprouts with Crispy Bacon (page 191)**
WEDNESDAY	Mediterranean Salmon Salad	Beetroot and Fennel Soup Brussels Sprouts with Crispy Bacon	Sage-Braised Chicken Legs (page 228)*** Puréed Parsnips (page 196) Sautéed Market Greens (page 183)
THURSDAY	Three-Herb Beef Patties	Puréed Parsnips Sautéed Market Greens	Sage-Braised Chicken Legs Brussels Sprouts with Crispy Bacon Rainbow Roasted Root Vegetables (page 188)
FRIDAY	Garlic-Sage Chicken Patties	Sautéed Market Greens Rainbow Roasted Root Vegetables	Coconut Amino–Marinated Salmon (page 237) Cauliflower 'Fried Rice' (page 200) Rosemary Grilled Asparagus (page 195)
SATURDAY	Garlic-Sage Chicken Patties	Rainbow Roasted Root Vegetables Rosemary Grilled Asparagus	Coconut Amino–Marinated Salmon Cauliflower 'Fried Rice'

*Thaw two servings of soup **Thaw one serving of soup ***Halve recipe

ALTERNATE 4-WEEK MEAL PLAN

	WEEK 1	WEEK 2
PANTRY ITEMS	**SATURDAY**	**SATURDAY**
solid cooking fat of your choice (lard, tallow, duck fat, etc.) coconut oil extra-virgin olive oil coconut concentrate ground ginger ground turmeric ground sage ground cinnamon bay leaves sea salt coconut flour kalamata olives capers apple cider vinegar coconut aminos shredded coconut flakes	900 g grass-fed beef mince 900 g free-range chicken thigh, minced 450 g wild-caught salmon 450 g grass-fed sirloin steak 1 bunch broccolini or broccoli 1 large head cauliflower 2 bunches dark leafy greens (kale, chard, spring greens) 1 bunch chard 1.3 kg carrots 680 g parsnips 1 courgette (zucchini) 1 sweet potato 180 g mushrooms fresh sage (2 bunches) 2 oranges fresh chives fresh mint fresh rosemary fresh thyme	900 g grass-fed beef brisket or stewing beef 450 g grass-fed beef mince 1 head savoy cabbage 1 large butternut squash 1.3 kg carrots 900 g beetroots 3 parsnips 1 swede 4 courgettes (zucchini) 1–2 avocados 2 firm pears 90 g mushrooms fresh flat-leaf parsley fresh rosemary fresh sage fresh thyme
KEEP IN STOCK	**WEDNESDAY**	**WEDNESDAY**
onions red onions fresh garlic fresh ginger lemons BPA-free tinned salmon BPA-free tinned tuna **HAVE READY** fermented vegetables (page 37) bone broth (page 34) garlic 'mayo' (page 127)	450 g free-range chicken breast 1 bunch curly-leafed kale 900 g sweet potatoes 1 head lettuce 1 bunch radishes 2 cucumbers 225 g jicama fresh mint fresh flat-leaf parsley 45 g raisins	450 g wild-caught salmon 2 bunches dark green leafy (kale, spring greens, chard) 1–2 bunches spinach 900 g parsnips 2 carrots 900 g asparagus 1 cucumber 1 avocado 1 orange fresh flat-leaf parsley fresh rosemary

SHOPPING LIST

WEEK 3	WEEK 4
SATURDAY	**SATURDAY**
900 g grass-fed beef mince 900 g free-range chicken thigh, minced 450 g free-range chicken breast 1.3 kg butternut squash 1.3 kg beetroots 1 large fennel bulb 2 heads of lettuce 1 bunch kale 4 carrots 2 cucumbers 1 avocado fresh dill fresh flat-leaf parsley fresh rosemary fresh sage (2 bunches) fresh thyme	450 g sole, flounder or John Dory 6 rashers sugar-free bacon 1 bunch curly-leafed kale 680 g brussels sprouts 1 head lettuce 2 carrots 1 beetroot 3 cucumbers 45 g mushrooms 1 avocado fresh mint fresh flat-leaf parsley fresh tarragon
WEDNESDAY	**WEDNESDAY**
900 g sweet potatoes 1 bunch celery 1 head cauliflower 4 courgettes (zucchini) 2 portobello mushrooms fresh rosemary	450 g free-range chicken legs and thighs 450 g wild-caught salmon 2 bunches dark leafy greens (kale, spring greens, chard) 900 g asparagus 1 head cauliflower 1.3 kg parsnips 6 carrots 3 beetroots 1 swede 1 courgette (zucchini) 270 g mushrooms 1 orange fresh chives fresh rosemary fresh sage (2 bunches)

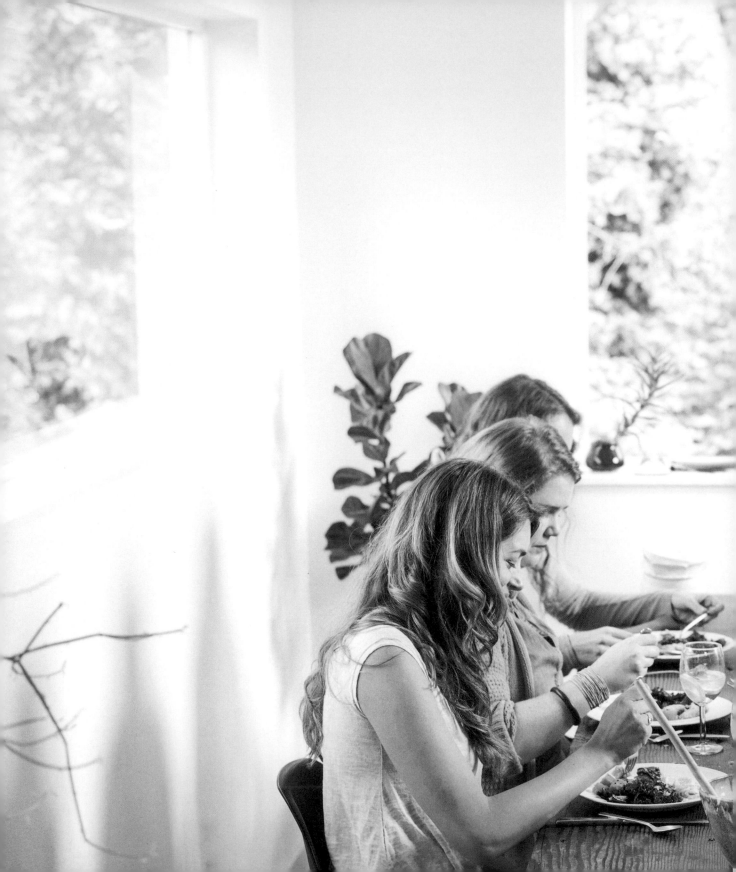

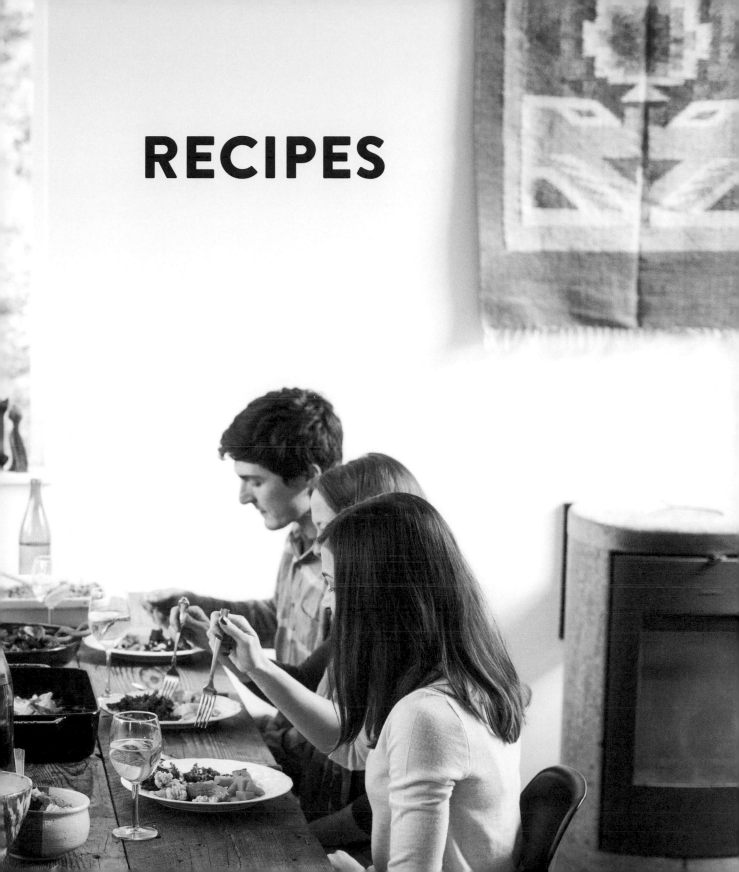

RECIPES

APPETISERS + SNACKS

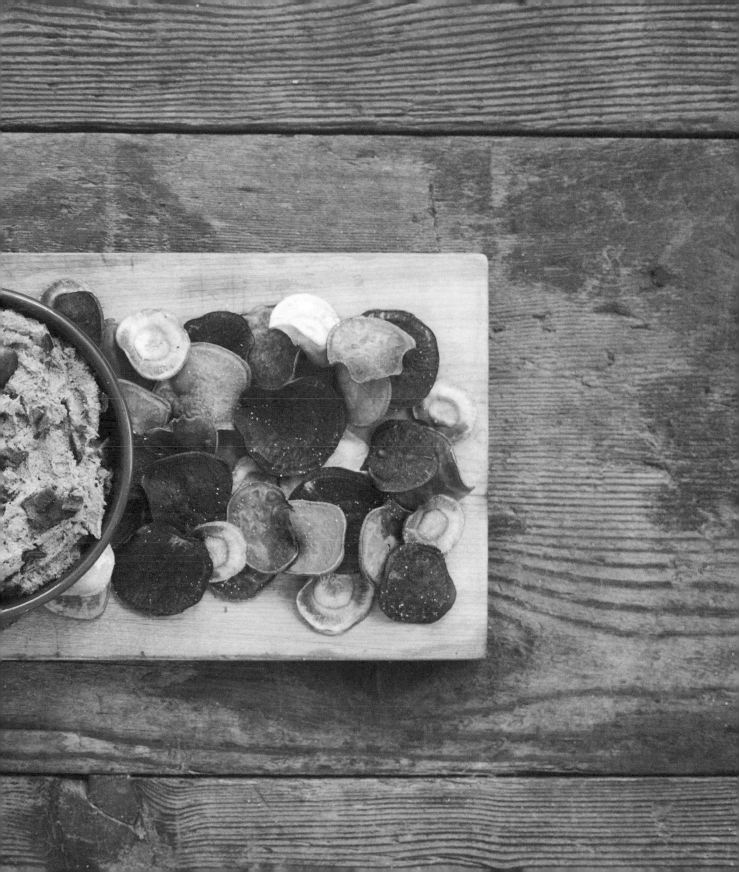

CRISPY KALE CHIPS

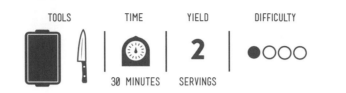

TOOLS | TIME | YIELD | DIFFICULTY

30 MINUTES | 2 SERVINGS | ●○○○

1 bunch kale, stems removed, leaves chopped into 5 cm pieces

2 tablespoons coconut oil, melted

Sea salt

1 Preheat the oven to 150°C.

2 Place the kale in a large bowl and coat with the coconut oil, stirring to cover completely.

3 Arrange the kale pieces on two or three baking trays, making sure to leave plenty of space between the pieces.

4 Bake for 20 minutes or until crispy. Remove from the sheet and add salt to taste. Let cool completely (the chips will crisp more as they cool) and serve.

Note: The trick to crispy kale chips is to make sure the kale is completely dry when it goes into the oven, and to salt it only after baking, as the salt will draw moisture out of the leaves, resulting in soggy chips.

Storage: Keeps sealed in an airtight container at room temperature for several days.

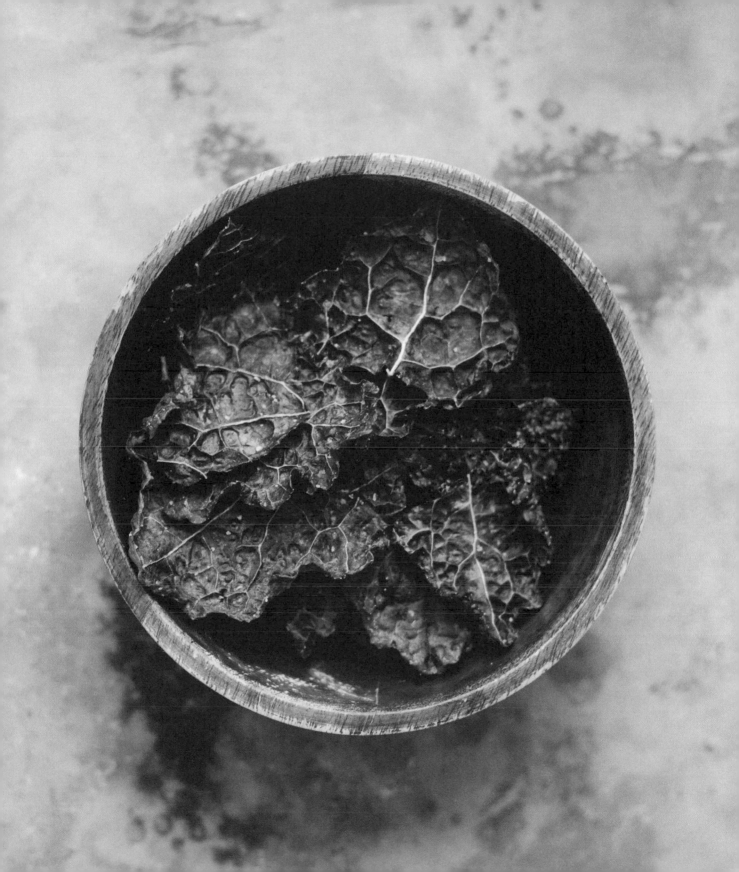

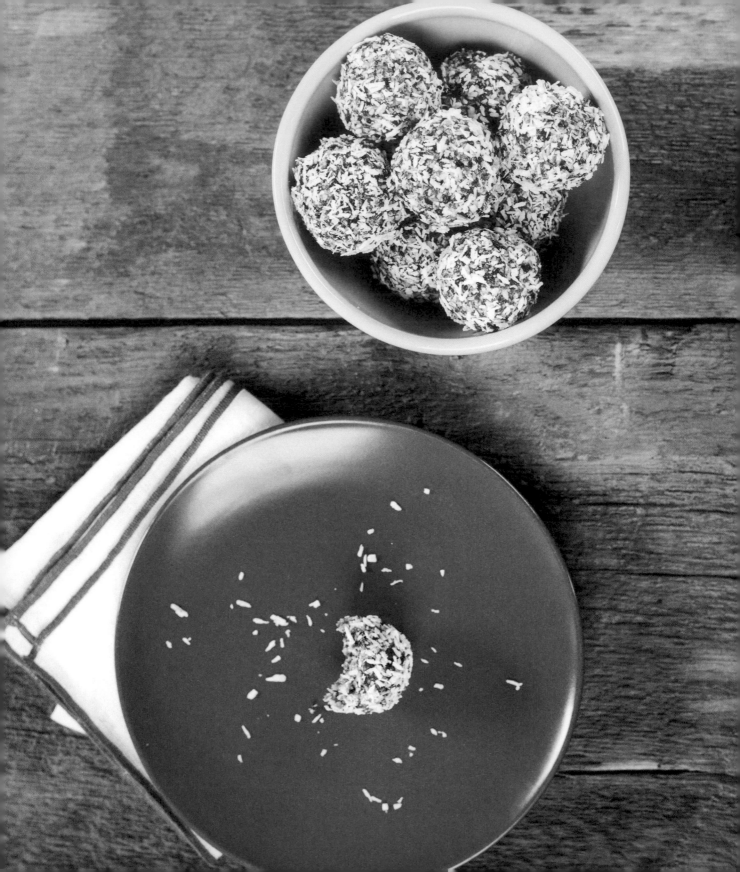

FIG ENERGY BITES

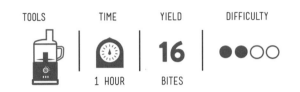

1 HOUR   **16** BITES   ●●○○

370 g unsulphured dried figs

130 g fine shredded coconut, divided (unsweetened)

80 ml coconut oil, melted

¼ teaspoon ground cinnamon

Pinch of sea salt

1 Place the figs, 100 g of the coconut, coconut oil, cinnamon and salt in a food processor and pulse on and off until a thick paste forms (you may have to stop and scrape the sides of your food processor a couple of times).

2 Form into 2.5 cm balls, then roll them in the reserved 30 g of shredded coconut.

3 Refrigerate for at least 30 minutes to let the coconut oil set.

Note: Feel free to play around with the dried fruit in this recipe—dates, dried apples and apricots are all good substitutions for the figs.

Storage: Keeps for a week or two stored in the refrigerator. Also freezes well.

NECTARINE, ROCKET AND PROSCIUTTO WRAPS

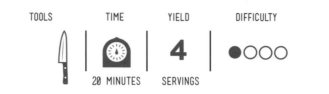

TOOLS | TIME | YIELD | DIFFICULTY

20 MINUTES | 4 SERVINGS | ●○○○

2 nectarines, pitted and cut
   into eighths
35 g rocket leaves
115 g thinly-sliced prosciutto

1 Hold a slice of nectarine in your hand and place a few sprigs of rocket alongside it. Use a partial slice of prosciutto to hold them together by wrapping it around the nectarine, about halfway up. The little tufts of rocket will stick out of the top.

2 Arrange on a serving platter.

Variation: Use any other stone fruit in place of the nectarine—peaches, plums and apricots all work well for this recipe.

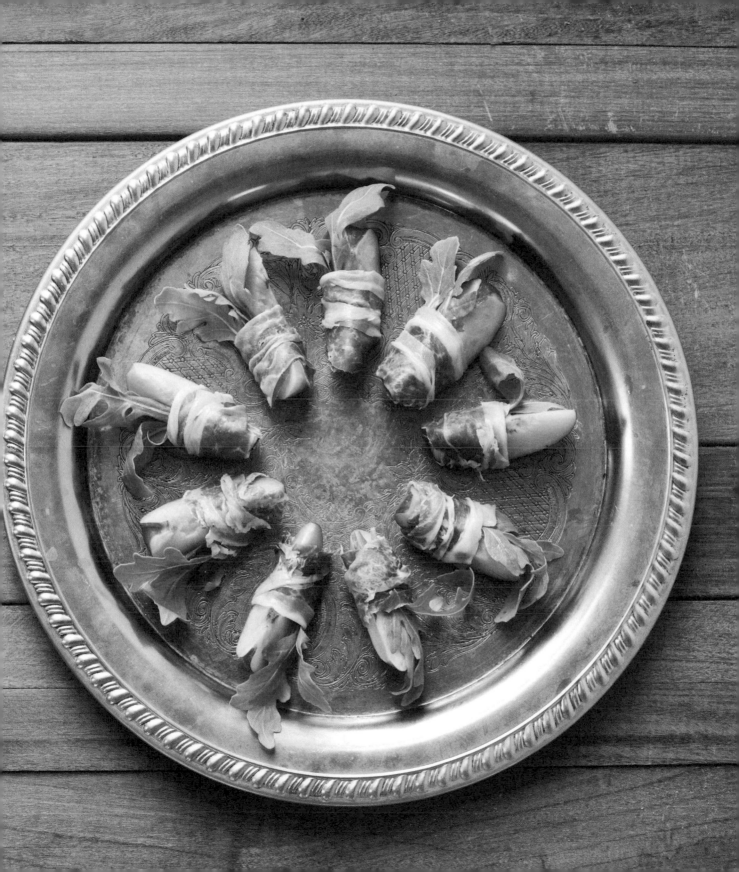

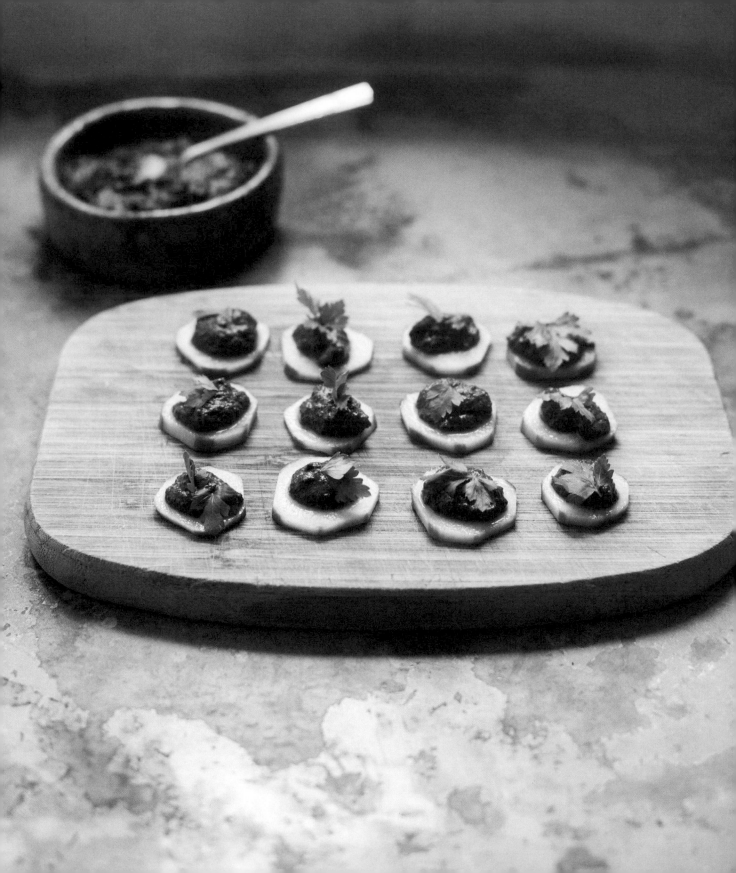

OLIVE TAPENADE

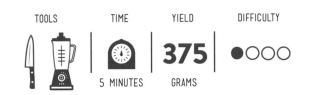

TOOLS | TIME | YIELD | DIFFICULTY

375

5 MINUTES | GRAMS | ●○○○

150 g pitted kalamata olives

2 tablespoons capers

3 tablespoons extra-virgin
olive oil

2 cloves garlic

small handful fresh flat-leaf
parsley leaves

Slices of fresh carrot, cucumber,
or Rainbow Root Vegetable
Chips (page 95)

1 Place the olives, capers, olive oil, garlic and parsley in a blender or food processor. Blend on low speed for a few seconds, until a thick paste forms. If it is too thick, add an extra tablespoon of olive oil.

2 Serve with fresh vegetable slices or root vegetable chips and a few extra parsley leaves.

Variation: For a fancier preparation, serve a spoonful of tapenade on a cucumber slice, topped with a sprig of parsley.

Storage: Keeps in the refrigerator for several days.

BACON–BEEF LIVER PATÉ WITH ROSEMARY AND THYME

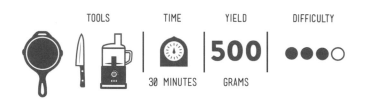

TOOLS	TIME	YIELD	DIFFICULTY
	30 MINUTES	**500** GRAMS	●●●○

6 rashers of sugar-free bacon

1 small onion, minced

4 cloves garlic, minced

450 g grass-fed beef liver, rinsed, dried and sliced into 5–7.5 cm pieces

2 tablespoons minced fresh rosemary leaves

2 tablespoons minced fresh thyme

80 ml coconut oil, melted

½ teaspoon sea salt

Fresh herbs, for garnish

Slices of fresh carrot or cucumber, for serving

1 Cook the bacon in a cast-iron frying pan, flipping as needed. Cook until crispy. Transfer to a paper towel-lined plate to cool, reserving the fat in the pan.

2 Add the onion to the pan and cook for about 5 minutes, stirring, on medium–high heat. Add the garlic and cook for a minute, then add the liver, rosemary and thyme. Cook 2 to 5 minutes per side, or until the liver is no longer pink in the center. Set aside to cool for a few minutes.

3 Transfer the mixture into a blender* or food processor with the coconut oil and sea salt. Process until it forms a thick paste.

4 Place the paté into a small bowl. Chop the cooled bacon into fine pieces (reserve some for garnish if you like) and combine with the paté.

5 Garnish with some reserved crispy bacon and the fresh herbs and serve with vegetable slices.

*Note: This recipe is difficult to make in a standard blender—you really need a high-powered machine with a tamper for best results.

Storage: Keeps in the refrigerator for several days. Also freezes well.

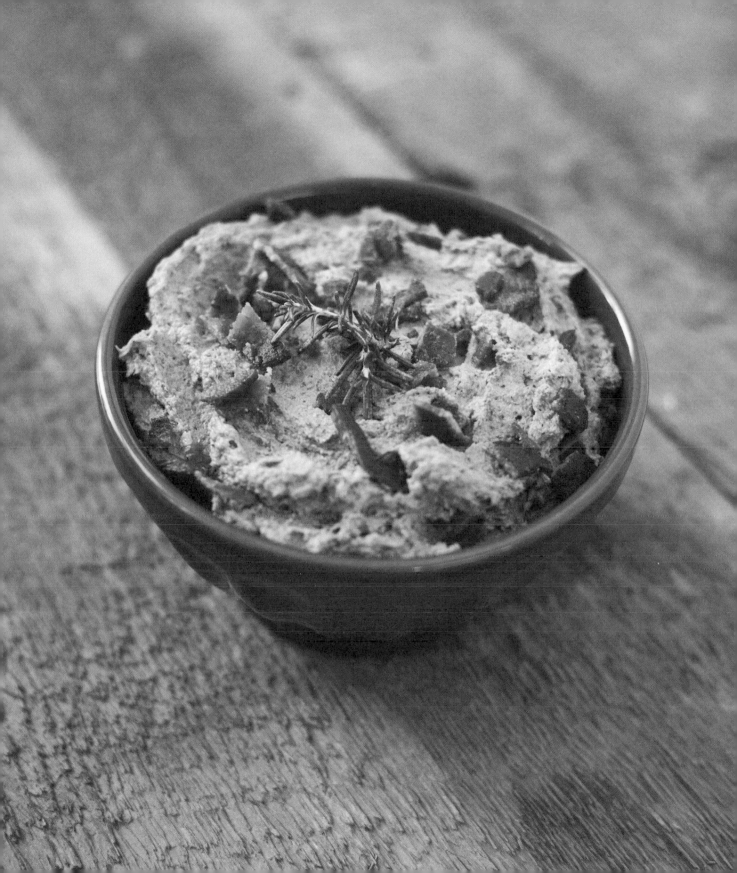

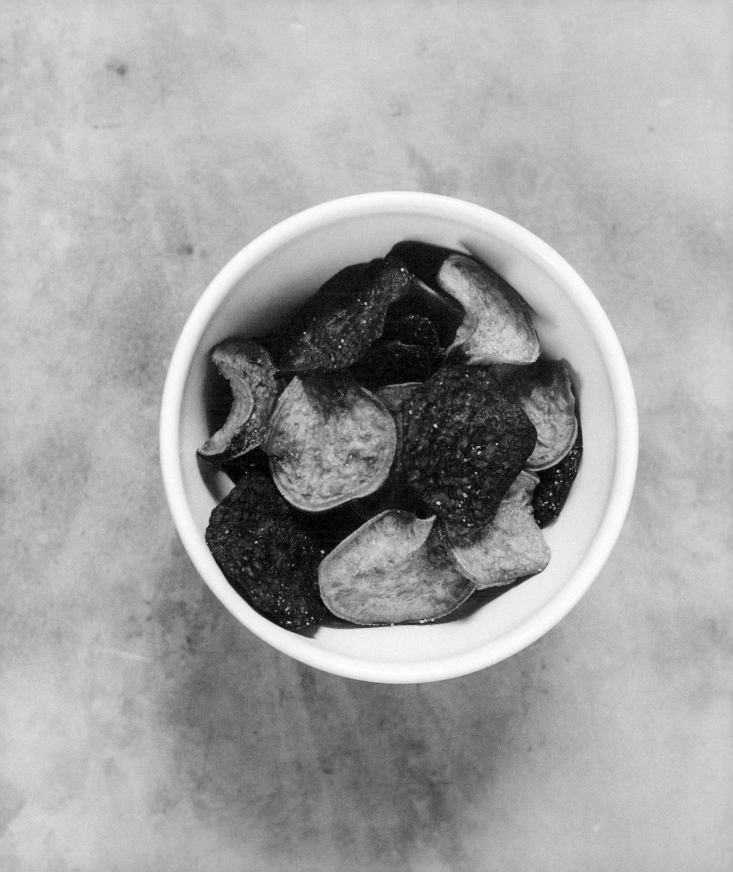

RAINBOW ROOT VEGETABLE CHIPS

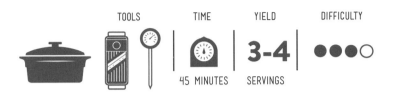

TOOLS · TIME · YIELD · DIFFICULTY

45 MINUTES

3-4 SERVINGS

●●●○

335 g root vegetables, thinly
   sliced*
Solid cooking fat, for frying
Sea salt

1 Attach a deep-fry thermometer to the side of a deep, heavy pot. Add enough solid cooking fat to make about 4 cm of melted fat. Heat over medium heat until the fat reaches 180°C. You want to be careful not to get the oil too hot, as it will burn the chips.

2 Fry the vegetables in batches by type, as they have different cooking times depending on how much moisture they contain. When you first drop the vegetable slices in the oil they will bubble like crazy; after a minute or two of cooking, they will start to bubble less and puff up in the middle. At this point, carefully turn them, and continue cooking until the bubbling dies down a lot. When it is apparent they don't have any moisture left, they are finished cooking.

3 Using a slotted spoon, carefully transfer the chips to a paper towel-lined plate and sprinkle with salt to taste. Bring the oil temperature back up to 180°C and continue in this fashion until all the chips are cooked.

*Note: I recommend using a mandoline to get consistently thin slices for this recipe. Your chips will cook more evenly, and chopping will be a lot less work! I also recommend using a deep-fry thermometer to ensure that the oil temperature stays consistent.

Variations: You can use any type of root vegetables for this recipe: sweet potato, carrots, beetroots, parsnips, turnips and swede all work well. Using a variety makes for a colourful batch!

Storage: Keeps sealed in an airtight container at room temperature for several days.

PARSLEY-GARLIC DIP

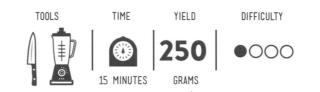

TOOLS	TIME	YIELD	DIFFICULTY
	15 MINUTES	250 GRAMS	●○○○

60 g fresh flat-leaf parsley
   leaves
40 g chopped red onion
2 cloves garlic
10 kalamata olives, pitted
¼ teaspoon sea salt
125 ml extra-virgin olive oil
1 lemon, juiced
   (about 2 tablespoons)
Slices of fresh carrot or
   cucumber, or Rainbow Root
   Vegetable Chips (page 95)
   or Crispy Kale Chips
   (page 84)

1 Combine all ingredients in a high-powered blender or food processor. Blend on low speed for a few seconds until a thick paste forms.

2 Serve on raw vegetable slices or with root vegetable or kale chips.

Storage: Keeps for several days in a sealed container in the refrigerator.

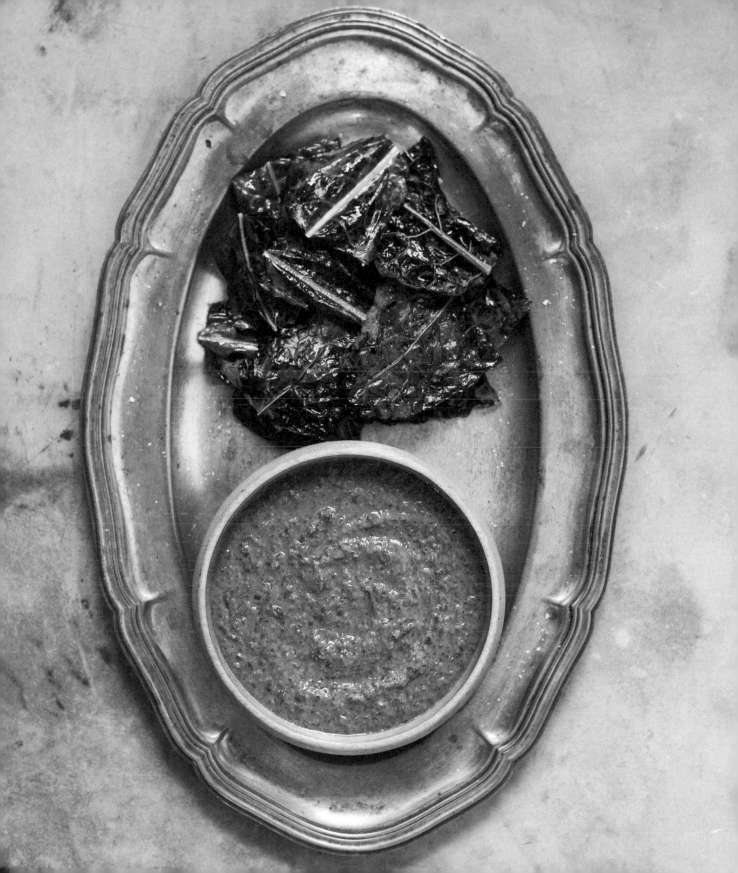

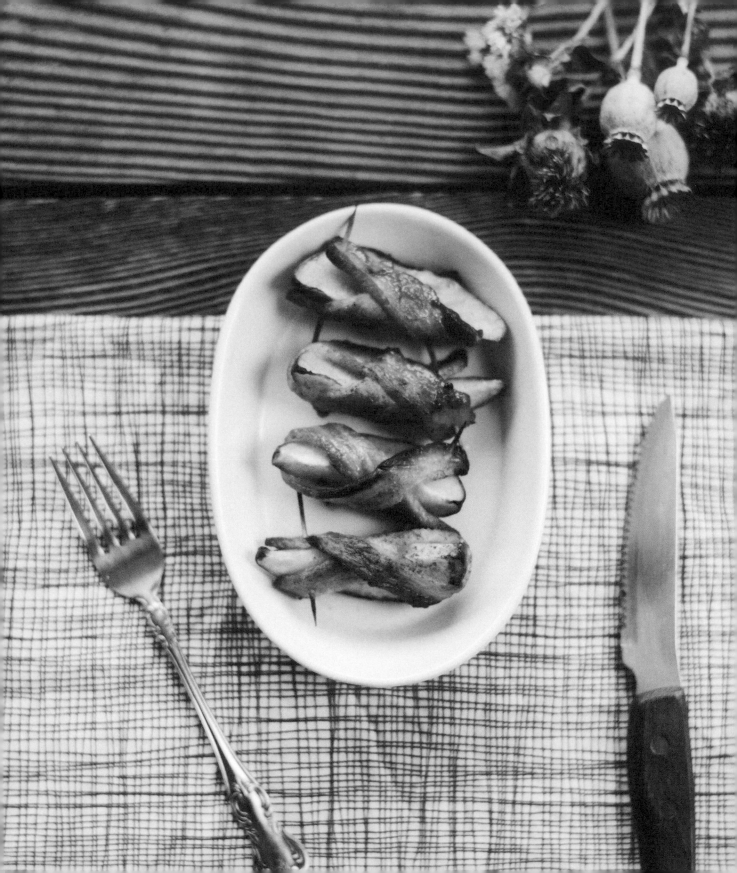

BACON-WRAPPED PEARS

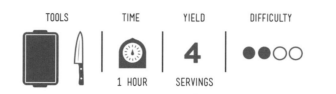

TOOLS | TIME | YIELD | DIFFICULTY

4 SERVINGS

1 HOUR

●●○○

6 rashers of thick, sugar-free bacon, cut in half lengthwise
2 ripe pears, cored and sliced into 6 pieces each
Toothpicks
Ground cinnamon

1 Preheat the oven to 180°C.

2 Wrap each pear slice in bacon, making a figure eight and securing the loose ends of bacon with a toothpick. Dust lightly with cinnamon and place on a rimmed baking tray.

3 Bake for 35 to 40 minutes, or until the bacon browns and the pears are cooked throughout.

4 Let cool for 10 minutes and serve warm.

Variation: Substitute apples for the pears or switch the flavour profile by using ground ginger instead of cinnamon. If you use apples, be advised they may need longer to cook.

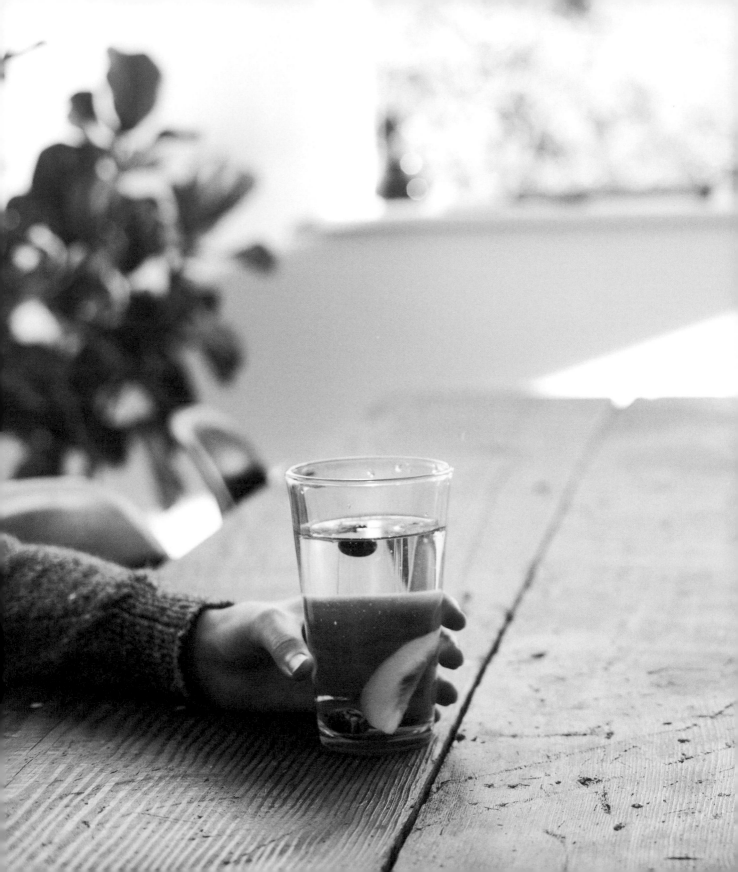

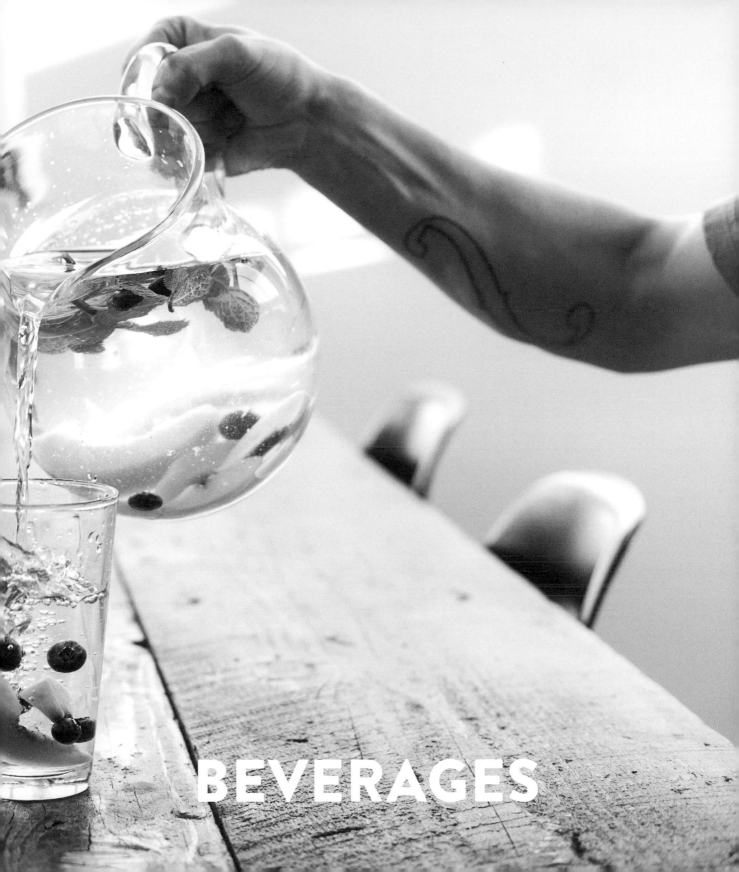

BEVERAGES

COCONUT MILK CHAI

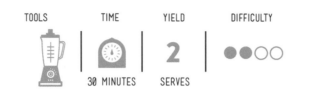

TOOLS | TIME | YIELD | DIFFICULTY

30 MINUTES

2 SERVES

55 g fine shredded coconut
(unsweetened)
1 whole vanilla pod (optional)
¾ teaspoon ground cinnamon
4 cm piece ginger, peeled
4 dates, pitted
500 ml boiling water

You will also need:
Muslin

1 Place all ingredients in a high-powered blender and blend on high for a minute or two, until thoroughly combined.

2 Let cool for 15 to 20 minutes.

3 When the liquid is cool enough to handle, strain it through a fine muslin or nut milk bag; squeeze the contents to yield the maximum amount of liquid.

4 Enjoy iced or reheat in a saucepan.

Storage: Keeps in the refrigerator for several days, but the fat may separate—heat gently and whisk to recombine.

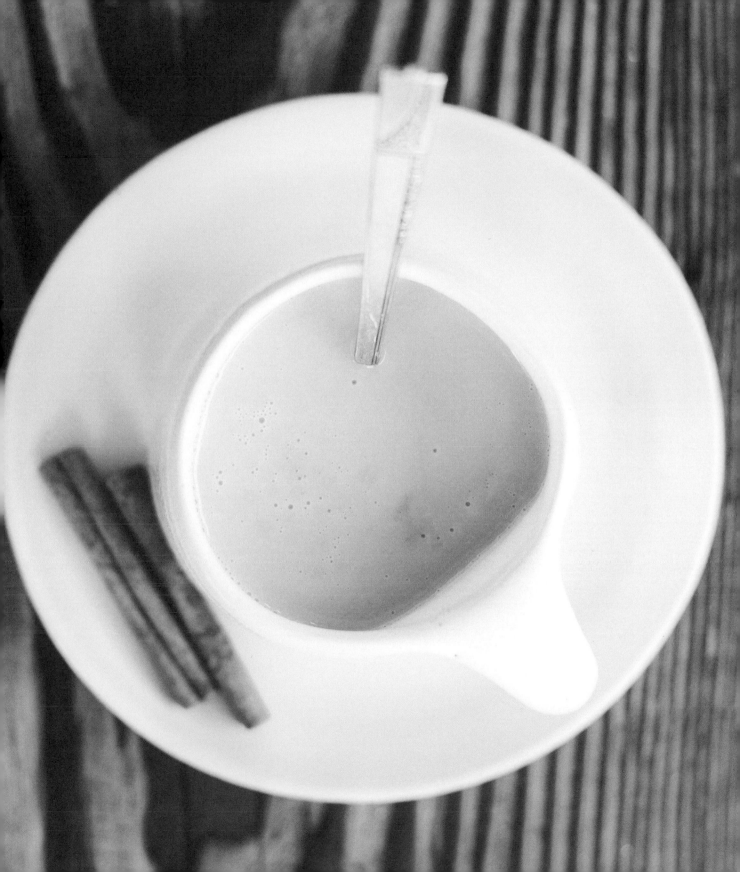

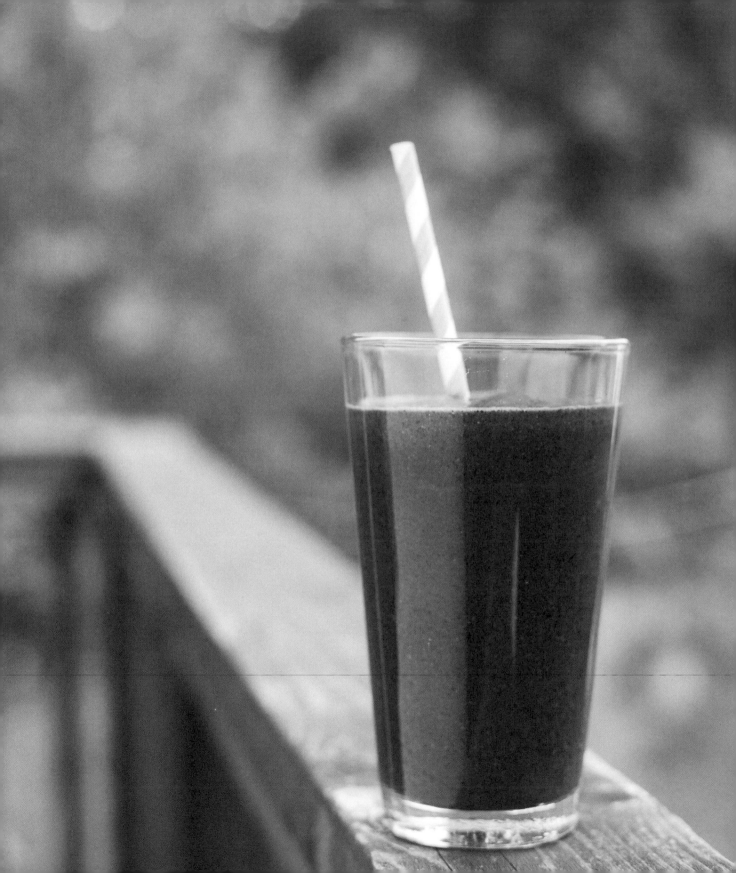

BANANA-BLUEBERRY GREEN SMOOTHIE

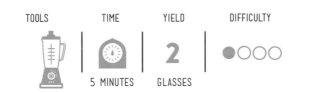

TOOLS | TIME | YIELD | DIFFICULTY

5 MINUTES | 2 GLASSES

1 medium banana
40 g fresh spinach leaves
70 g blueberries, frozen
2 tablespoons Coconut
Concentrate (page 45)
185 ml filtered water
Ice cubes (optional)

1 Place all ingredients in a blender and blend until well incorporated.

2 If you prefer a thicker or colder drink, add a few ice cubes and blend again. Serve immediately.

Variation: You can substitute kale, chard or other leafy greens for the spinach, or other types of berries for the blueberries. Don't skip the banana or coconut concentrate! They make the drink thick and deliciously creamy.

RASPBERRY CREAM SMOOTHIE

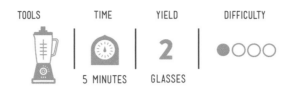

TOOLS	TIME	YIELD	DIFFICULTY
	5 MINUTES	2 GLASSES	●○○○

1 banana
100 g frozen raspberries
2 tablespoons Coconut
   Concentrate (page 45)
185 ml filtered water
Ice cubes (optional)

1 Place all ingredients in a blender and blend until well incorporated.

2 If you prefer a thicker or colder drink, add a few ice cubes and blend again. Serve immediately.

Variation: Use blueberries, strawberries or blackberries instead of raspberries.

MANGO DREAM SMOOTHIE

TOOLS	TIME	YIELD	DIFFICULTY
	5 MINUTES	2 GLASSES	●○○○

130 g frozen mango pieces
1 banana
185 ml filtered water
2 tablespoons coconut oil
1 tablespoon chopped fresh mint
   leaves (optional)
Ice cubes (optional)

1 Place all ingredients in a blender and blend until well incorporated.

2 If you prefer a thicker or colder drink, add a few ice cubes and blend again. Serve immediately.

Variation: Use frozen pineapple instead of mango.

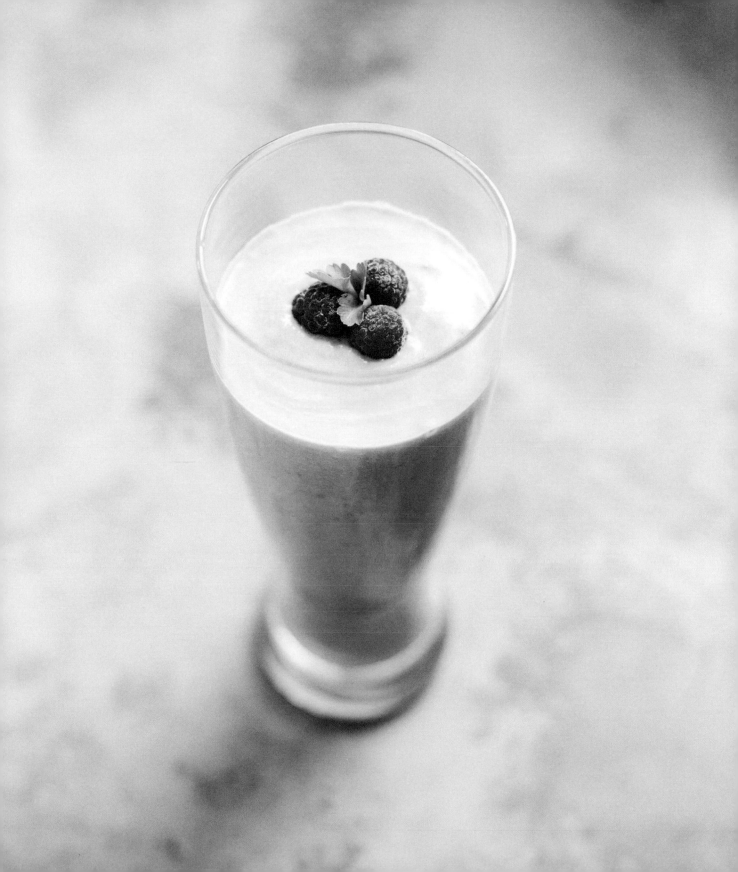

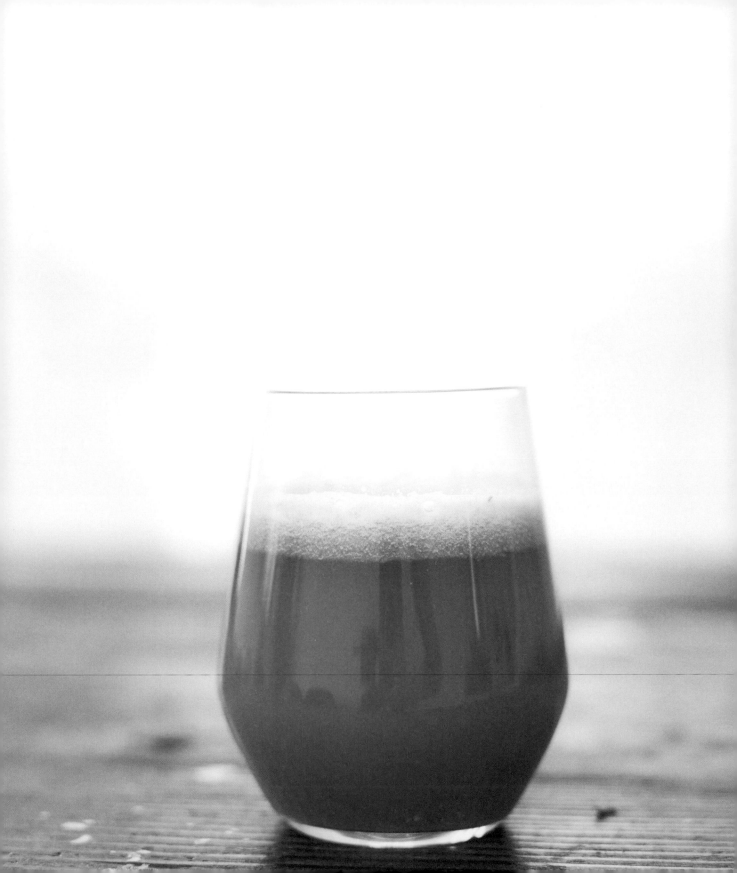

GREEN POWER JUICE

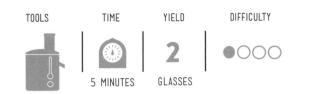

TOOLS	TIME	YIELD	DIFFICULTY
	5 MINUTES	2 GLASSES	●○○○

1 small pear, cored
4 large leaves kale
A handful of fresh mint leaves
2 large cucumbers, peeled
1 lemon, juiced (about 2
    tablespoons)

1 Feed the pear, kale and mint leaves into a juicer; end with the cucumbers to help ensure that the kale and mint get pushed through.

2 Add the lemon juice, stir, and serve immediately.

Variation: Substitute apple for the pear, or for a less-sweet version, use celery instead of pear.

GINGER BOOST JUICE

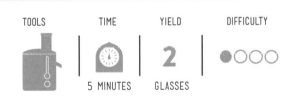

TOOLS	TIME	YIELD	DIFFICULTY
	5 MINUTES	2 GLASSES	●○○○

1 large cucumber, peeled
3 celery stalks
A handful of fresh flat-leaf
    parsley leaves
2.5 cm piece ginger, peeled
2 medium carrots, peeled

1 Feed the cucumber, celery, parsley and ginger into a juicer; end with the carrots to help push all the ingredients through. Stir and serve immediately.

Variation: Substitute half of a beetroot for the carrots.

INFUSED WATER

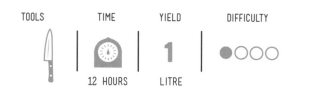

TOOLS	TIME	YIELD	DIFFICULTY
	12 HOURS	1 LITRE	●○○○

Acidic Fruit:

Lemon
Lime
Grapefruit
Orange

Sweet Fruit/Vegetable:

Blueberry
Raspberry
Peach
Mango
Pineapple
Cherry
Cucumber

Herb:

Mint
Lavender
Sage
Rosemary
Thyme

1 Add a slice of acidic fruit, a handful of sweet fruit or vegetable, and a couple sprigs of your herb to 1 litre of filtered water.

2 Let sit overnight in the refrigerator. You can enjoy the infused water immediately, but the longer you let the fruit and herbs infuse the water, the more the flavour will intensify.

3 Serve and enjoy!

Note: Feel free to use fresh or frozen fruit for this recipe. Also, don't be afraid to try some things I have not listed here—these are my favorites, but the sky is the limit when it comes to how many herb and fruit combinations you can come up with!

Storage: Keeps in the refrigerator for several days.

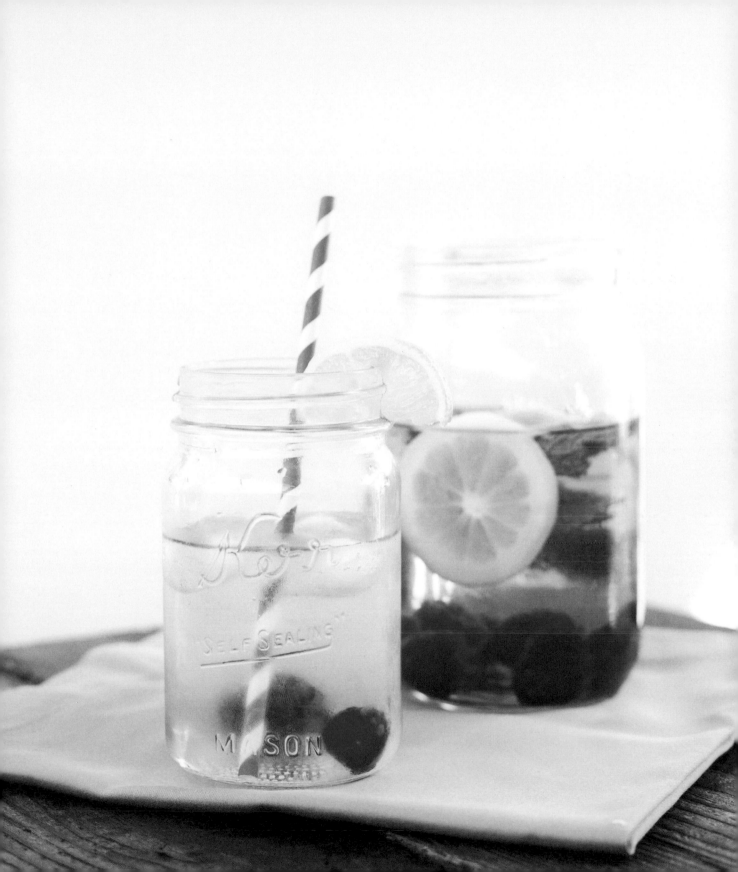

DRESSINGS + SAUCES

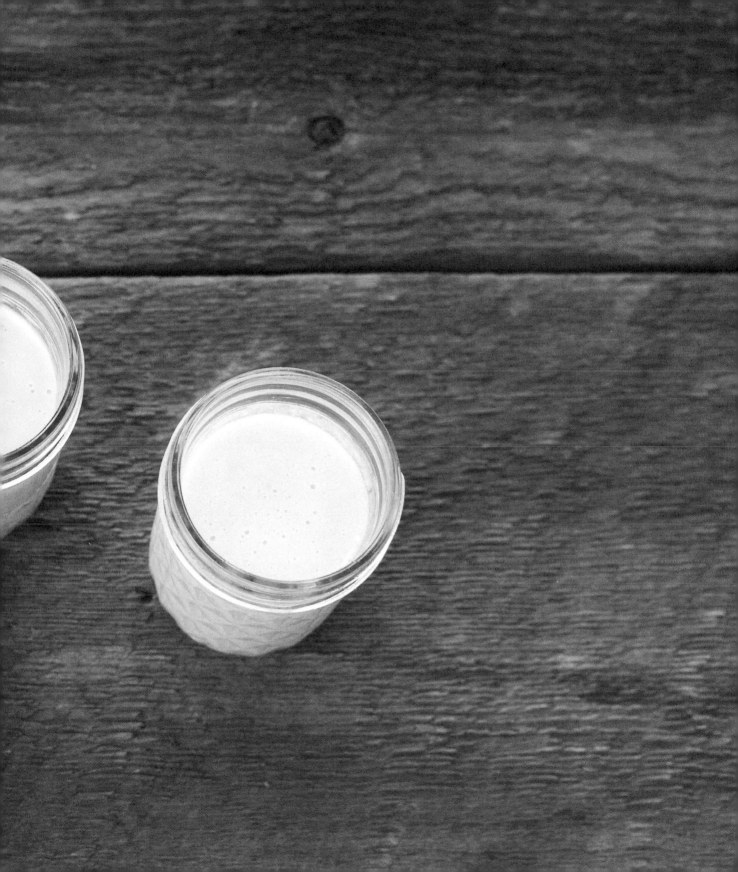

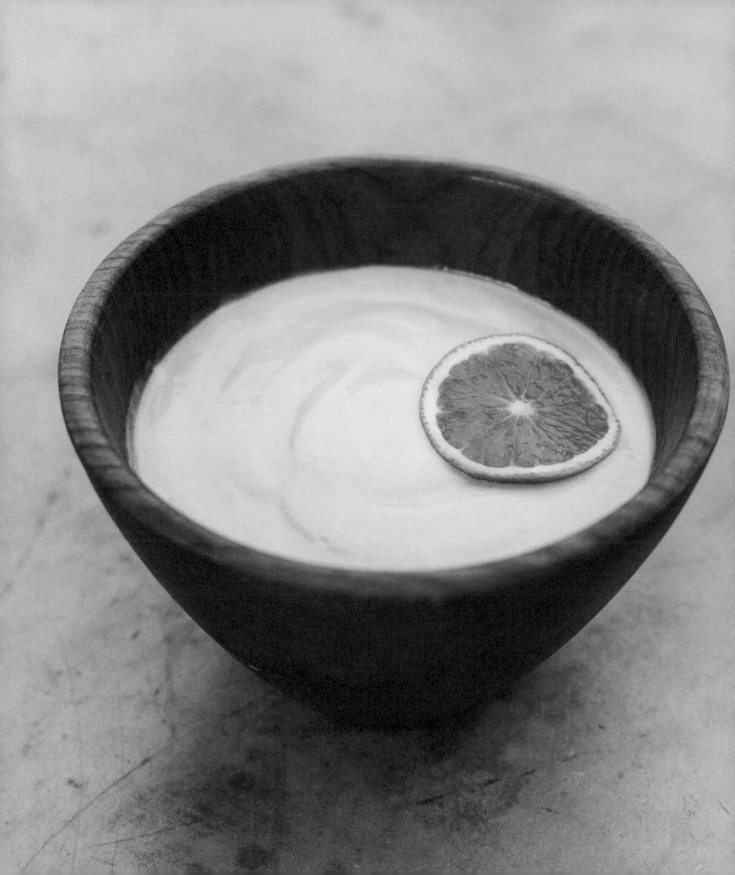

CITRUS-AVOCADO DRESSING

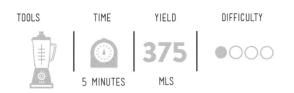

TOOLS | TIME 5 MINUTES | YIELD 375 MLS | DIFFICULTY ●○○○

1 avocado, peeled and destoned
1 orange, juiced
   (about 4 tablespoons)
1 lemon, juiced
   (about 2 tablespoons)
60 ml extra-virgin olive oil
60 ml filtered water,
   plus more as needed
1 teaspoon apple cider vinegar
¼ teaspoon ground ginger
¼ teaspoon sea salt

1 Combine all ingredients in a blender and mix until well incorporated.

2 If dressing is too thick, add more water one tablespoon at a time until desired consistency is reached.

Storage: Keeps for a day, sealed, in the refrigerator.

OLIVE-AVOCADO DRESSING

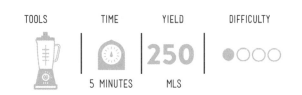

TOOLS | TIME 5 MINUTES | YIELD 250 MLS | DIFFICULTY ●○○○

1 avocado, peeled and destoned
80 ml extra-virgin olive oil
80 ml filtered water
2 teaspoons apple cider vinegar
½ lemon, juiced
   (about 1 tablespoon)
¼ teaspoon sea salt

1 Combine all ingredients in a blender and mix for a few seconds until well incorporated.

2 If dressing is too thick, add water one tablespoon at a time until desired consistency is reached.

Storage: Keeps for a day, sealed, in the refrigerator.

RASPBERRY VINAIGRETTE

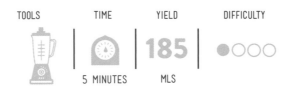

TOOLS	TIME	YIELD	DIFFICULTY
	5 MINUTES	185 MLS	●○○○

125 ml extra-virgin olive oil

30 g raspberries (fresh or frozen)

2 tablespoons apple cider vinegar

¼ teaspoon ground ginger

¼ teaspoon sea salt

1 Combine all ingredients in a blender and mix for a few seconds until well incorporated.

Variation: Feel free to use other fruit instead of the raspberries here—plums or figs would be wonderful substitutions.

Storage: Keeps well in the refrigerator for several days. Shake or stir before using.

BLOOD ORANGE VINAIGRETTE

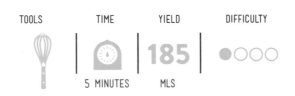

TOOLS	TIME	YIELD	DIFFICULTY
	5 MINUTES	185 MLS	●○○○

2 blood oranges, juiced
(about 4 tablespoons)

125 ml extra-virgin olive oil

2 teaspoons ume plum vinegar

¼ teaspoon ground ginger

1 Combine all the ingredients in a small bowl and whisk to incorporate.

Variation: Use apple cider or coconut vinegars instead of ume plum; but if you do, make sure to add sea salt to taste, as those vinegars are not as salty as the plum. Regular oranges also work well if you can't find blood oranges.

Storage: Keeps for several days, sealed, in the refrigerator.

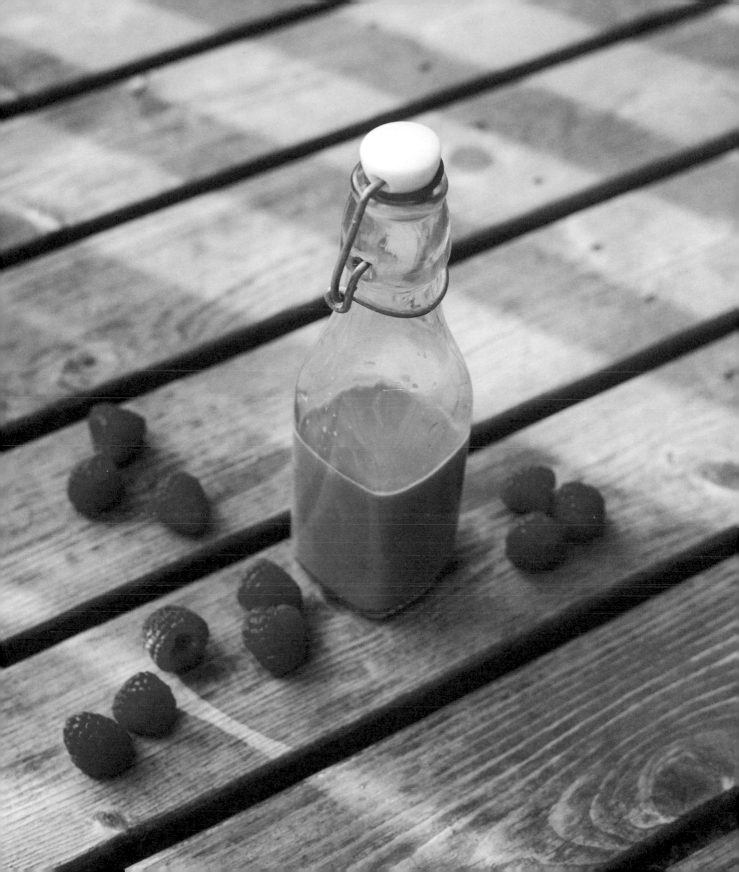

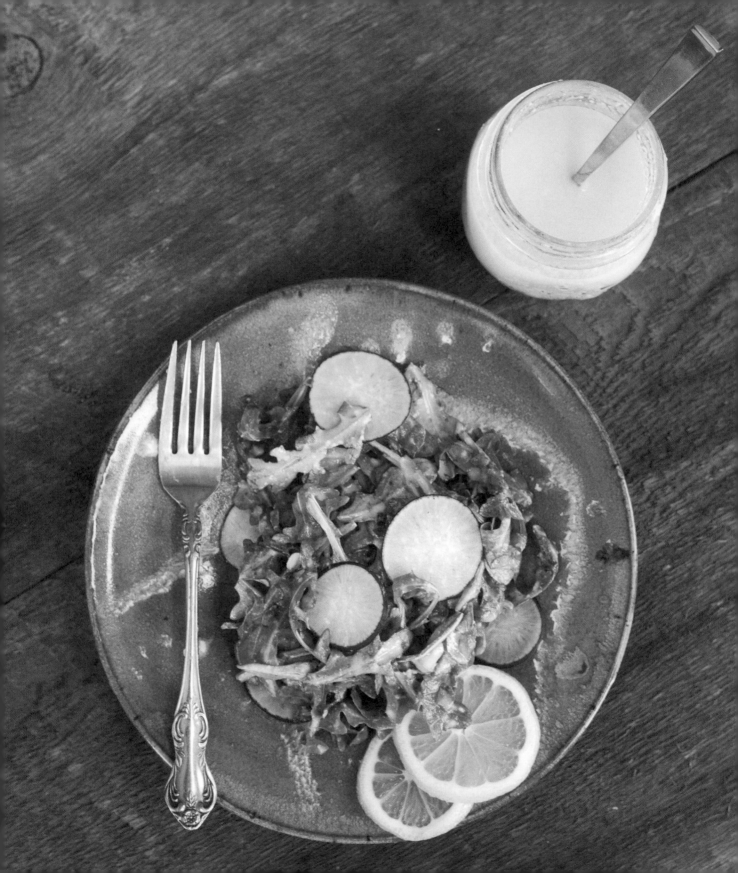

CAESAR SALAD DRESSING

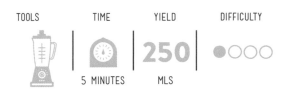

TOOLS	TIME	YIELD	DIFFICULTY
	5 MINUTES	250 MLS	●○○○

60 ml Coconut Concentrate
(page 45)*

125 ml filtered water or
coconut milk

80 ml extra-virgin olive oil

2 cloves garlic

1 lemon, juiced (about 2
tablespoons)

¼ teaspoon sea salt

2 anchovy fillets

1 Combine all ingredients in a blender and mix for a minute until
well incorporated.

2 If the dressing is too thick, add water one tablespoon at a time until desired
consistency is reached.

*Note: In order to measure the coconut concentrate, it is best to soften it in a warm
water bath before use as it is solid at room temperature.

Storage: This dressing keeps in the refrigerator for several days, but hardens.
Bring back to room temperature or warm slightly before using.

GINGER-LIME
COCONUT CREAM DRESSING

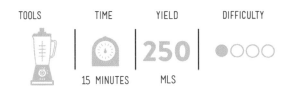

TOOLS	TIME	YIELD	DIFFICULTY
	15 MINUTES	250 MLS	●○○○

125 ml Coconut Concentrate
(page 45)*

125 ml filtered water

2 limes, juiced
(about 1 tablespoon)

1 teaspoon apple cider vinegar

1½ teaspoons minced ginger

¼ teaspoon sea salt

1 Combine all ingredients in a blender and mix for a minute until
well incorporated.

2 If the dressing is too thick, add water one tablespoon at a time until desired
consistency is reached.

*Note: In order to measure the coconut concentrate, it is best to soften it in a warm
water bath before use as it is solid at room temperature.

Storage: This dressing keeps in the refrigerator for several days, but hardens.
Bring back to room temperature or warm slightly before using.

APPLE CIDER VINAIGRETTE

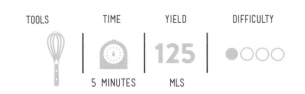

TOOLS	TIME	YIELD	DIFFICULTY
	5 MINUTES	125 MLS	●○○○

125 ml extra-virgin olive oil

2 tablespoons apple cider vinegar

¼ teaspoon ground ginger

¼ teaspoon sea salt

1 Combine the olive oil, vinegar, ginger and salt in a small bowl and whisk to incorporate.

Variation: This is a great basic vinaigrette recipe that adapts well to improvisation; you can add different fruits or herbs as you prefer. Try adding berries, stone fruit or various fresh herbs to create your own seasonal dressings.

Storage: Keeps well in the refrigerator for several days. Shake or stir before using.

GINGER PLUM VINAIGRETTE

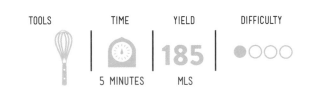

TOOLS	TIME	YIELD	DIFFICULTY
	5 MINUTES	185 MLS	●○○○

125 ml extra-virgin olive oil

1 tablespoon ume plum vinegar

1 lemon, juiced
(about 2 tablespoons)

1 teaspoon ground ginger

1 Combine the olive oil, vinegar, lemon juice and ginger in a small bowl and whisk to incorporate.

Variation: Use apple cider or coconut vinegar instead of ume plum—but if you do, make sure to add sea salt to taste, as those vinegars are not as salty as the plum.

Storage: Keeps well in the refrigerator for several days. Shake or stir before using.

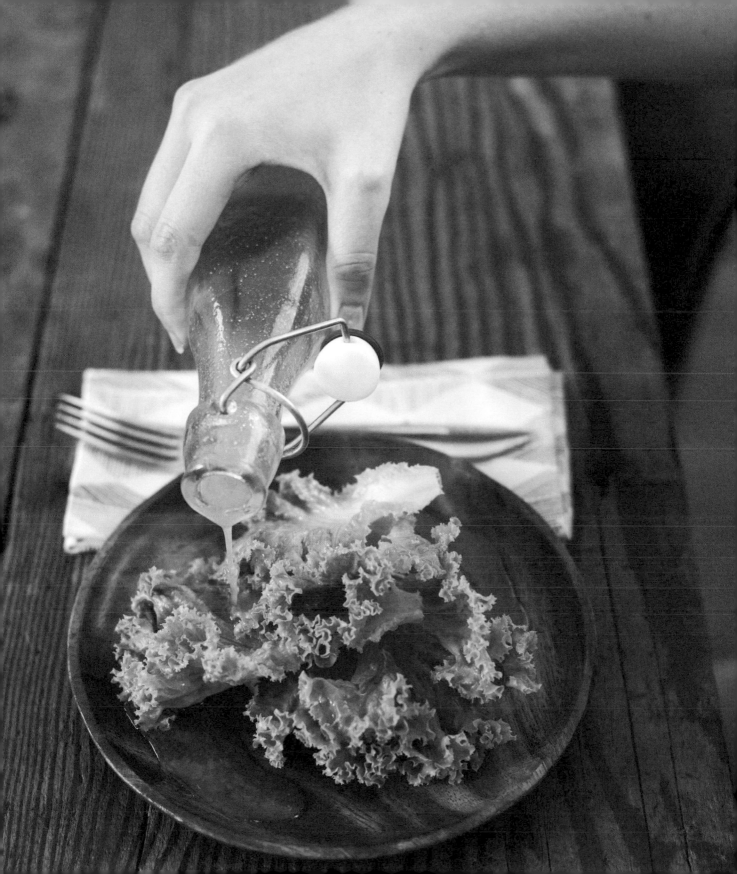

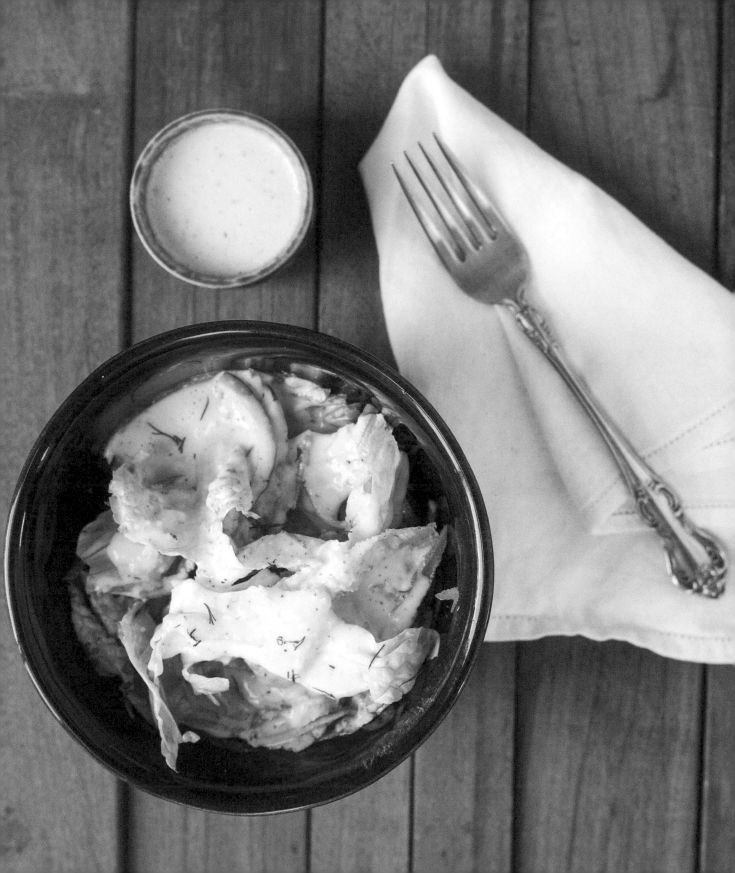

'RANCH' DRESSING

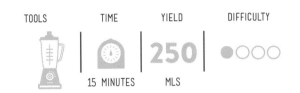

TOOLS	TIME	YIELD	DIFFICULTY
	15 MINUTES	250 MLS	●○○○

60 ml Coconut Concentrate
   (page 45)*
60 ml extra-virgin olive oil
125 ml filtered water or Creamy
   Coconut Milk (page 46)
½ lemon, juiced
   (about 1 tablespoon)
1 teaspoon apple cider vinegar
1 clove garlic
1 tablespoon chopped fresh dill
¼ teaspoon sea salt

1 Place all ingredients in a blender and mix until thoroughly combined.

2 If the dressing is too thick, thin it with water until the desired consistency is reached.

*Note: In order to measure the coconut concentrate, it is best to soften it in a warm water bath before use as it is solid at room temperature.

Storage: This dressing keeps in the refrigerator for several days, but hardens. Bring back to room temperature or warm slightly before using.

COCONUT-BASIL PESTO

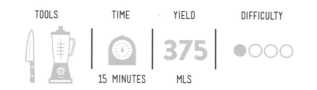

TOOLS	TIME	YIELD	DIFFICULTY
	15 MINUTES	375 MLS	●○○○

125 ml coconut water or
  filtered water
100 g fresh basil leaves
60 ml extra-virgin olive oil
4 cm piece ginger, peeled
  and chopped
2–3 cloves garlic, chopped
1 tablespoon ume plum
  vinegar
1 lemon, juiced
  (about 2 tablespoons)
A few sprigs of fresh mint

1 Place all ingredients into a blender and blend on high for 15 seconds, stopping to scrape the sides if needed. If you want a smoother pesto, continue to blend until desired consistency is reached.

Variation: Use apple cider or coconut vinegars and add sea salt to taste, as those vinegars are not as salty as the plum.

Storage: Keeps for a couple of days, sealed, in the refrigerator.

Serving Suggestions: Rainbow Roasted Root Vegetables (page 188), Sautéed Market Greens (page 183)

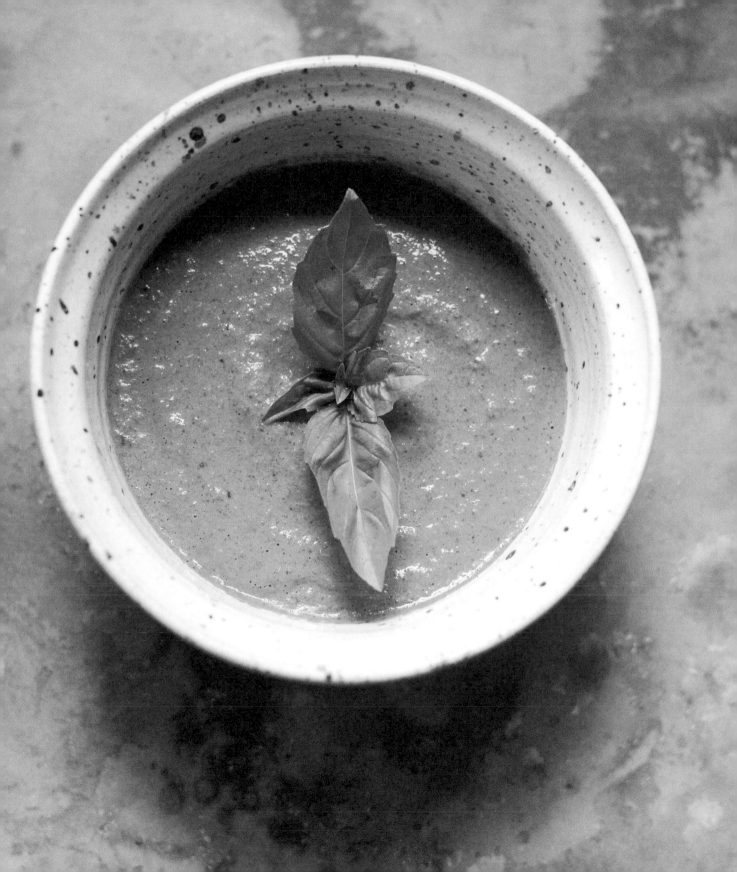

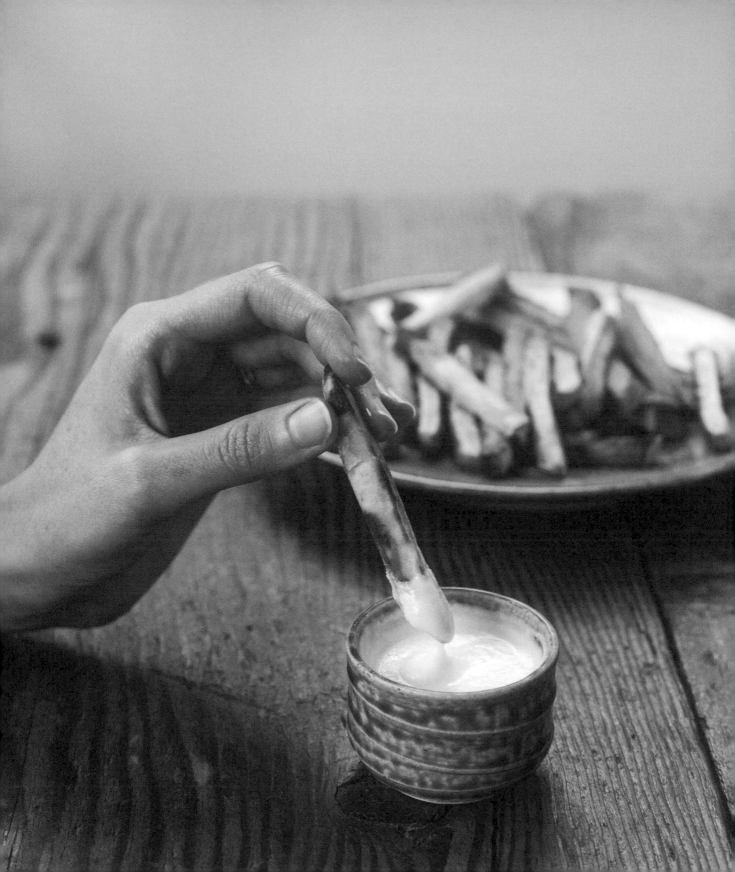

GARLIC 'MAYO'

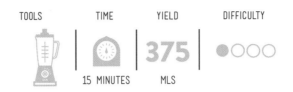

TOOLS | TIME | YIELD | DIFFICULTY

15 MINUTES | 375 MLS | ●○○○

125 ml Coconut Concentrate (page 45)*

125 ml filtered water, warm

60 ml extra-virgin olive oil

3 to 4 cloves garlic

¼ teaspoon salt

1 Place all of the ingredients in a blender and blend on high for a minute or two, until a thick sauce forms (when freshly made, it should resemble the consistency of conventional mayonnaise).

2 If the sauce is too thick, thin with water until the desired consistency is reached.

*Note: In order to measure the coconut concentrate, it is best to soften it in a warm water bath before use as it is solid at room temperature.

Storage: Keeps well in the refrigerator, but hardens. Let come to room temperature or warm to soften before using.

Serving Suggestions: Use to create dressings and sauces, as a topping for Three-Herb Beef Patties (page 262) or Garlic-Sage Chicken Patties (page 211), or as a dip for Rainbow Root Vegetable Chips (page 95).

GUACAMOLE

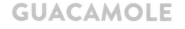

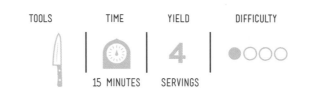

TOOLS | TIME | YIELD | DIFFICULTY

15 MINUTES | SERVINGS

2 large avocados, peeled, destoned and mashed

90 g finely chopped cucumber

40 g minced red onion

A small handful of chopped coriander

1 clove garlic, minced

1 lime, juiced (about ½ tablespoon)

1 tablespoon extra-virgin olive oil

1½ teaspoons apple cider vinegar

Sea salt

1 Combine all ingredients in a bowl and stir to combine. Season to taste with salt. Serve immediately.

Storage: Keeps for a day in the refrigerator.

Serving Suggestions: Serve on fresh vegetable slices, Rainbow Root Vegetable Chips (page 95), or as a condiment.

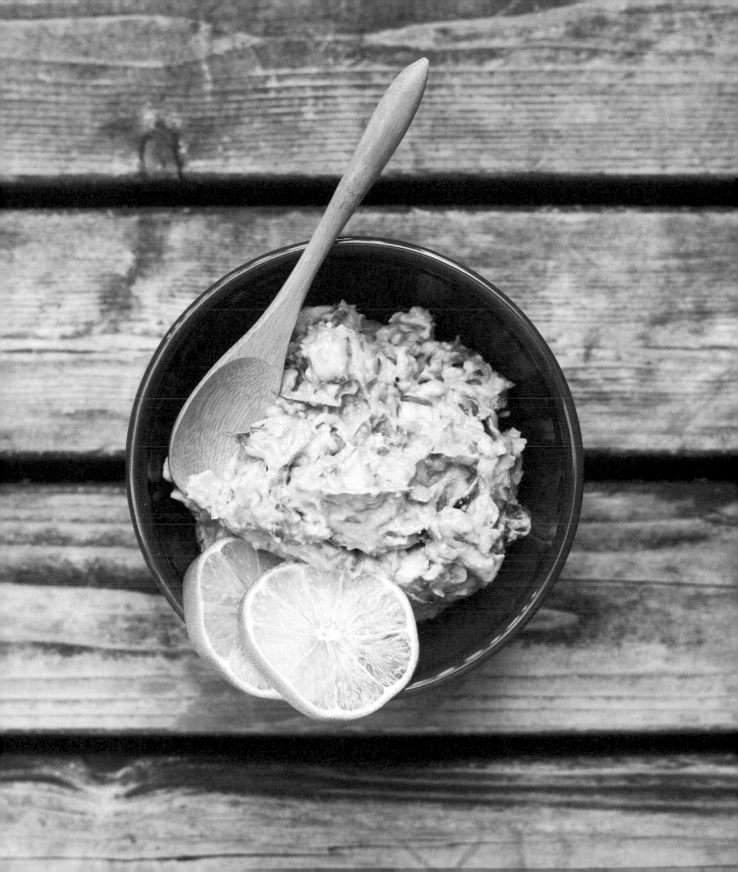

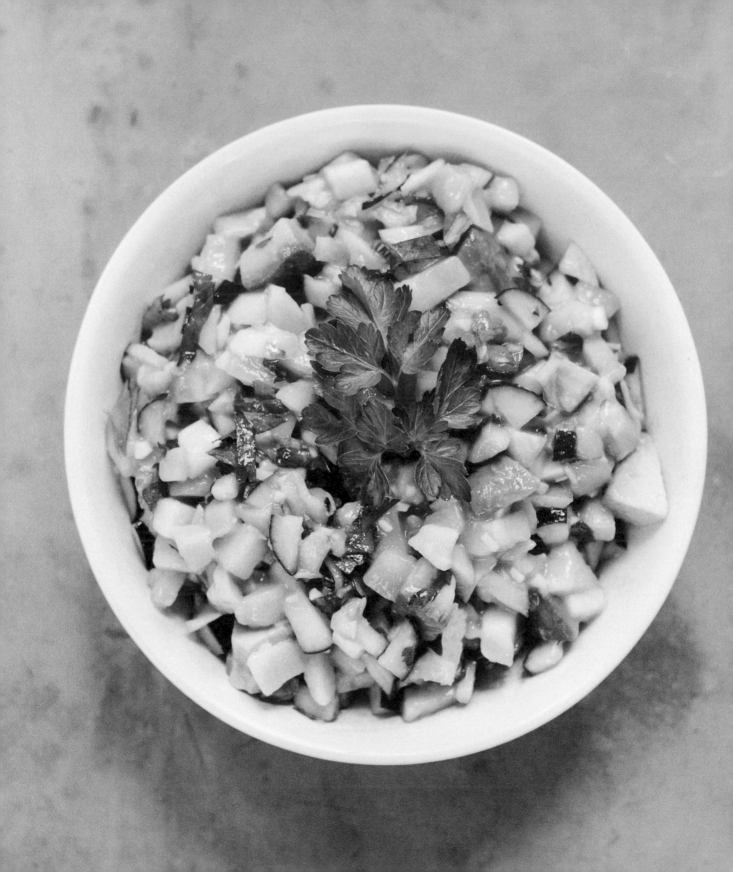

MANGO SALSA

TOOLS   TIME   YIELD   DIFFICULTY

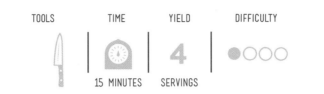

15 MINUTES   SERVINGS

1 large mango, peeled and diced

1 avocado, peeled, destoned
  and diced

½ small red onion, diced

1 cucumber, diced

1 bunch coriander, chopped

2 cloves garlic, minced

½ teaspoon sea salt

1 tablespoon olive oil

1 lime, juiced
  (about ½ tablespoon)

1 Combine all of the ingredients in a bowl and mix to incorporate.

Variation: Try substituting peaches, basil and lemon juice for the mango, coriander and lime juice.

Storage: Keeps in the refrigerator for several days.

Serving Suggestions: Serve in lettuce cups with Shredded Roast Beef (page 261), Coconut-Crusted Cod (page 241), on top of salads or as a condiment.

CHERRY BBQ SAUCE

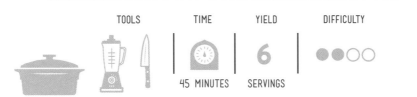

TOOLS	TIME	YIELD	DIFFICULTY
	45 MINUTES	6 SERVINGS	●●○○

2 tablespoons solid
   cooking fat

1 small onion, chopped

6 cloves garlic, minced

450 g pitted cherries, fresh
   or frozen, halved

60 ml maple syrup

3 tablespoons apple cider
   vinegar

1 teaspoon smoked sea salt

1 Heat the solid cooking fat in a saucepan on medium heat. When the fat has melted and the pan is hot, add the onion and cook for 5 minutes. Add the garlic and cook for another couple of minutes, stirring, until fragrant. Add the cherries, maple syrup, cider vinegar and smoked sea salt.

2 Cook uncovered over low heat for about 30 minutes, or until the mixture thickens considerably. Transfer to a blender and blend on high until smooth.

Variation: Feel free to use plums instead of cherries.

Storage: Keeps in the refrigerator for a week. Also freezes well.

Serving Suggestions: Lemon-Garlic Marinated Chicken (page 219), Herbed Dry-Rub Steak (page 265), Three-Herb Beef Patties (page 262), or instead of Garlic 'Mayo' on Portobello Burgers (page 274)

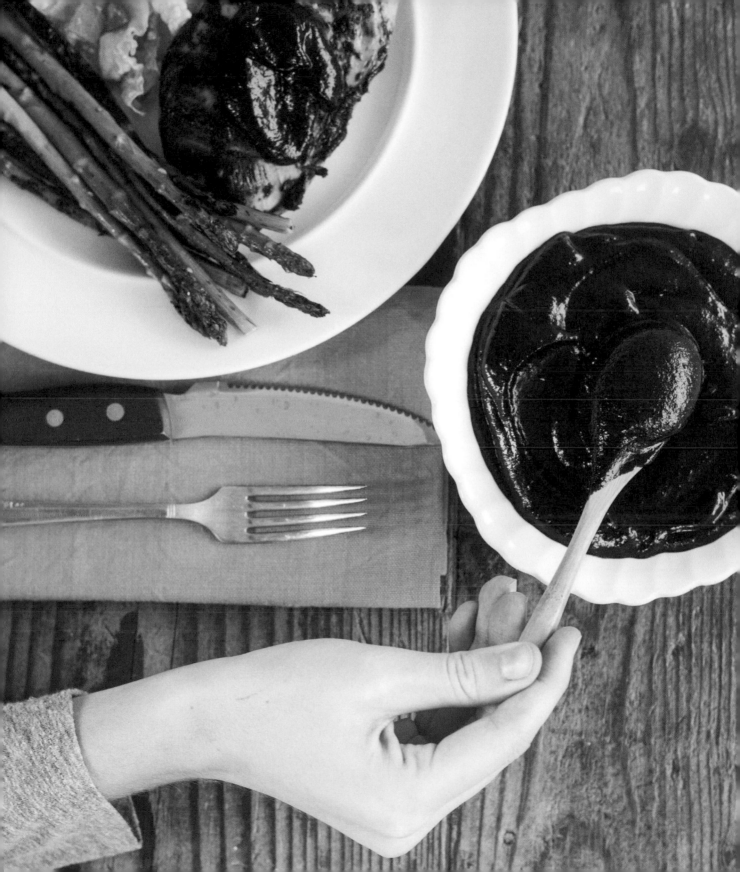

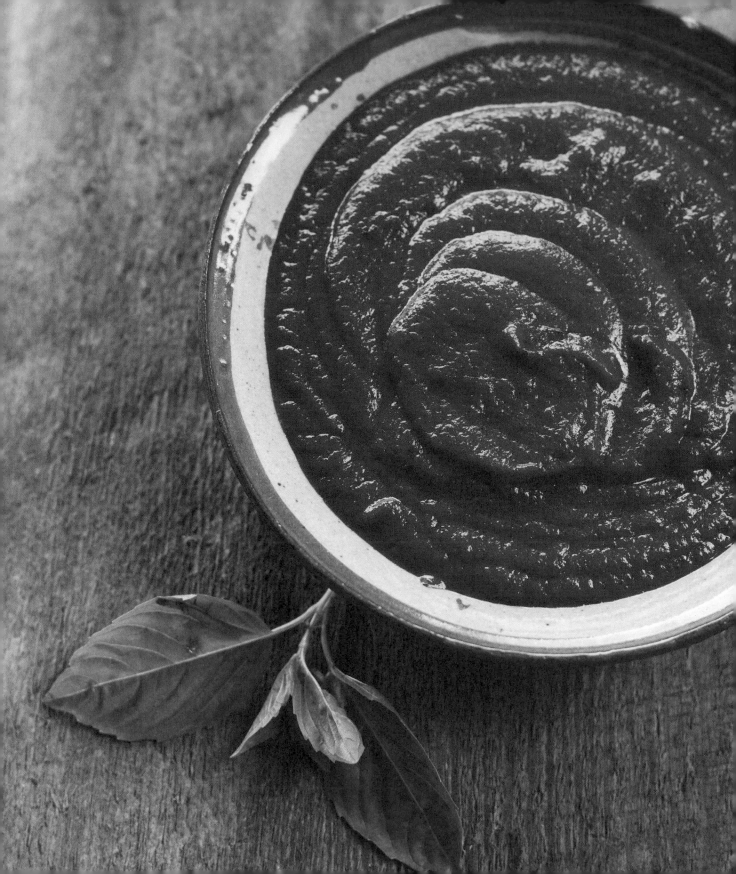

NOMATO SAUCE

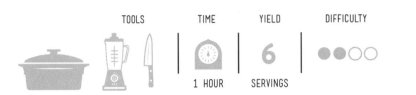

TOOLS	TIME	YIELD	DIFFICULTY
	1 HOUR	6 SERVINGS	●●○○

1 tablespoon solid cooking fat

1 large onion, chopped

4 cloves garlic, minced

2 medium beetroots, chopped

2 medium carrots, chopped

1 tablespoon fresh thyme

1 tablespoon fresh rosemary

250 ml Bone Broth (page 34)

1 teaspoon sea salt

A small handful of chopped fresh basil

1 Heat the cooking fat in a heavy-bottomed pot on medium heat. When the fat has melted and the pan is hot, add the onion and cook for about 5 minutes. Add the garlic and cook for another couple of minutes, stirring. Add the beetroot, carrot, thyme and rosemary and cook for another couple of minutes.

2 Add the bone broth and salt; bring to a boil. Lower the heat, then cover and simmer on low for 30 minutes, or until the vegetables are soft.

3 Carefully transfer the mixture to a blender and purée.

4 Add back to the pot and stir in the fresh basil, turning on the heat to cook for 5 more minutes.

Variation: Make this a meat sauce by adding 450 g of browned beef, lamb or pork mince just before adding the basil and simmering for another 10 minutes.

Storage: Keeps in the refrigerator for several days. Also freezes well.

Serving Suggestions: Serve on top of cooked spaghetti squash or courgette (zucchini) noodles. You can also add Three-Herb Meatballs (page 262) or Lamb Meatballs (page 277) to the sauce.

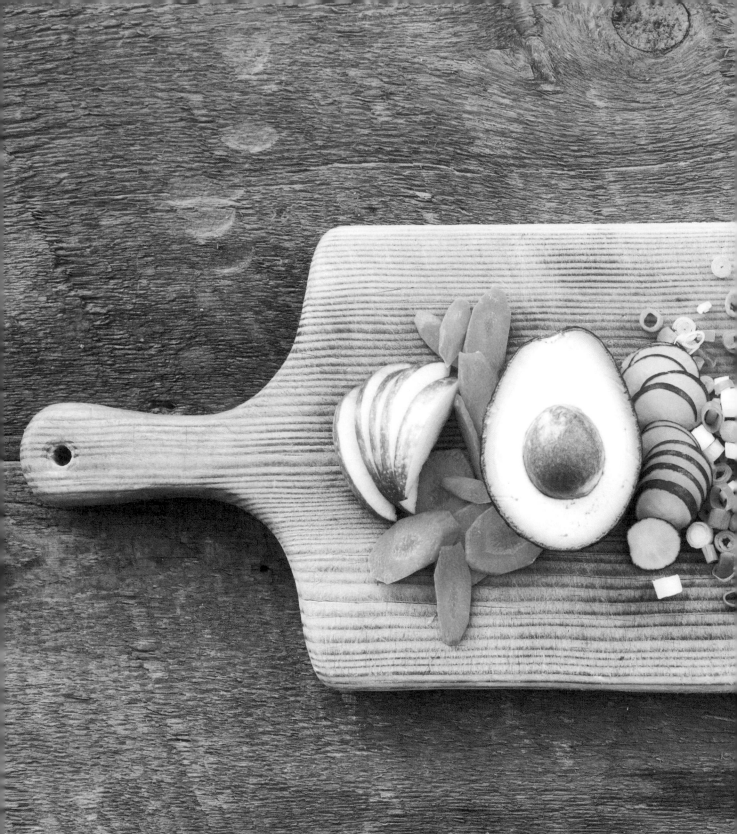

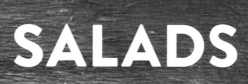

SALADS

EMERALD KALE SALAD

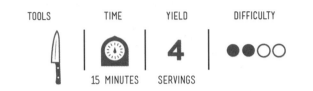

TOOLS   TIME   YIELD   DIFFICULTY

15 MINUTES   **4** SERVINGS   ●●○○

1 bunch curly kale, stems trimmed, leaves finely chopped

2 tablespoons olive oil

1 teaspoon sea salt

½ lemon, juiced (1 tablespoon)

40 g minced red onion

45 g finely chopped cucumber

1 Place the chopped kale in a large bowl; drizzle with olive oil and sprinkle with sea salt.

2 Massage the kale gently with your hands for 5 to 10 minutes, or until the tough fibres of the kale break down and soften somewhat.

3 Toss with the lemon juice, red onion and cucumber.

Storage: Keeps well in the refrigerator for several days.

Serving Suggestions: Mediterranean Salmon Salad (page 153), Garlic-Sage Chicken Patties (page 211), Curried Chicken Salad (page 224), Herb-Stuffed Trout (page 253), Three-Herb Beef Patties (page 262)

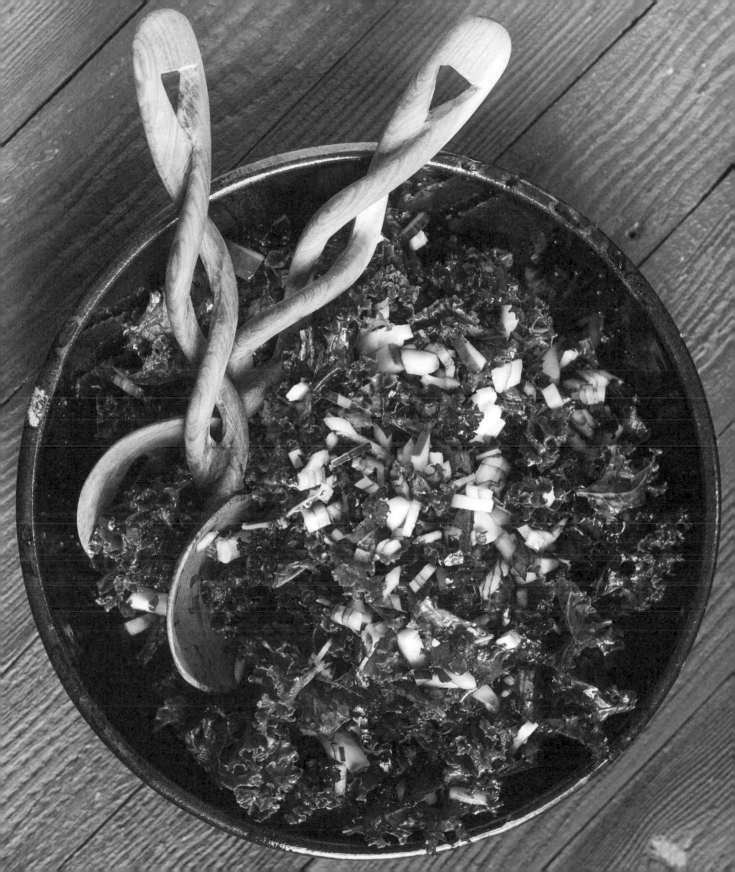

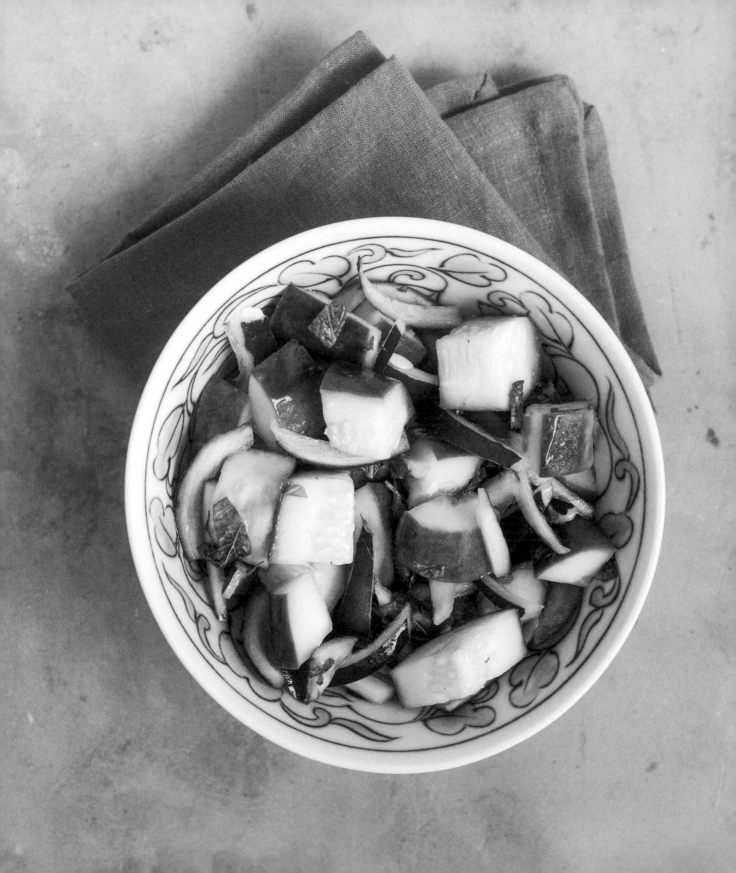

CUCUMBER-MINT SALAD

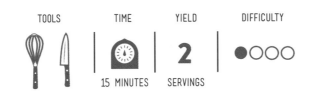

TOOLS   TIME   YIELD   DIFFICULTY

15 MINUTES   2 SERVINGS   ●○○○

2 large cucumbers, chopped

½ small red onion, thinly sliced

2 tablespoons chopped fresh parsley

2 tablespoons chopped fresh mint

2 tablespoons apple cider vinegar

3 tablespoons extra-virgin olive oil

Sea salt to taste

1 Combine the cucumbers, onion, parsley and mint in a bowl.

2 In a small bowl, whisk the apple cider vinegar, olive oil and sea salt.

3 Toss the dressing with the vegetables and serve.

Storage: Keep dressing separate and toss through the salad right before serving.

Serving Suggestions: Mediterranean Salmon Salad (page 153), Rosemary-Mint Lamb Patties (page 269), Lamb Chops with Rosemary-Plum Sauce (page 281), Radish and Jicama Tabbouli (page 142)

RADISH AND JICAMA TABBOULI

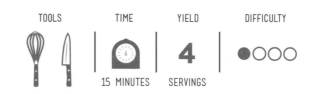

TOOLS   TIME   YIELD   DIFFICULTY

15 MINUTES   4 SERVINGS   ●○○○

1 bunch fresh flat-leaf parsley, chopped

1 bunch radishes, finely chopped

½ small jicama, peeled and finely chopped

2 carrots, finely chopped

1 cucumber, finely chopped

8 kalamata olives, pitted and minced

1 tablespoon minced fresh mint

60 ml extra-virgin olive oil

2 tablespoons apple cider vinegar

½ lemon, juiced (about 1 tablespoon)

Sea salt to taste

1 Combine the parsley, radishes, jicama, carrots, cucumber, olives and mint in a large bowl.

2 In a small bowl, whisk the olive oil, vinegar, lemon juice and salt.

3 Toss the dressing with the salad and serve.

Storage: Keeps in the refrigerator for several days.

Note: Jicama is also known as a Mexican yam or a Mexican turnip. If you can't track it down at your local market, crisp green apple, pear or even celery can be used in its place to give a similar crunch.

Serving Suggestions: Cucumber-Mint Salad (page 141), Rosemary-Mint Lamb Patties (page 269), Mediterranean Salmon (page 242), Salmon Salad with Olives and Cucumber (page 238), Curried Chicken Salad (page 224), Citrus-Ginger Marinated Salmon (page 237)

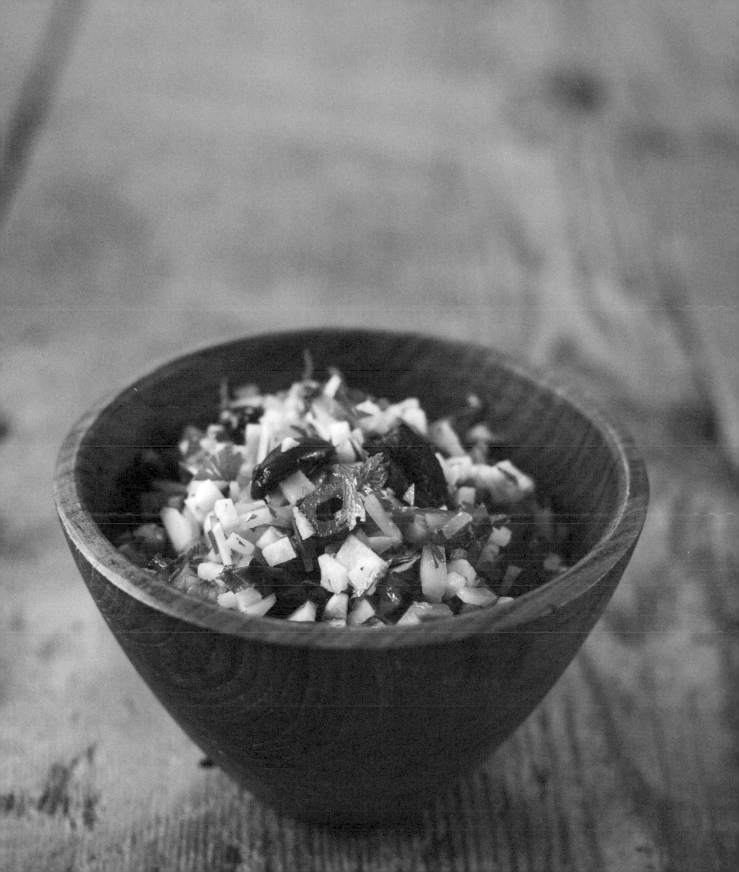

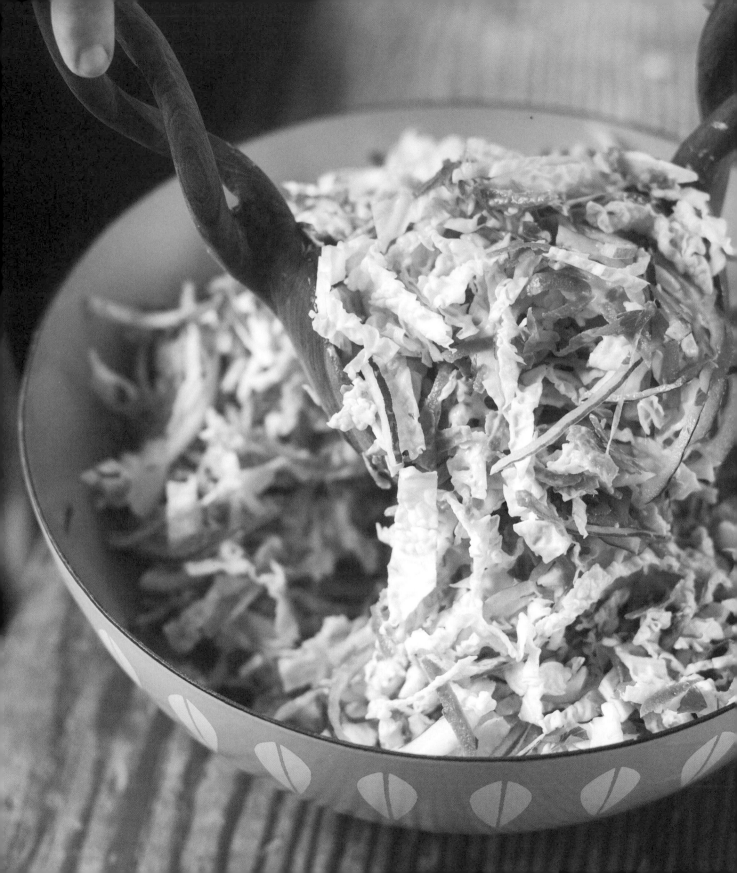

CABBAGE SLAW WITH OLIVE-AVOCADO DRESSING

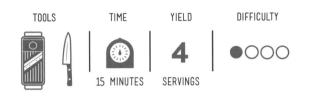

TOOLS   TIME   YIELD   DIFFICULTY

15 MINUTES   4 SERVINGS   ●○○○

1 small head Savoy cabbage, chopped (or substitute with other variety of green cabbage)

1 small red onion, thinly sliced

3 carrots, grated

1 handful chopped fresh flat-leaf parsley

250 ml Olive-Avocado Dressing (page 115)

1 In a large bowl, combine the cabbage, onion, carrots and most of the parsley.

2 Toss with the vegetables with the dressing and garnish with the remainder of the parsley.

Storage: Keep dressing separate and toss through the salad right before serving.

Serving Suggestions: Orange-Rosemary Duck (page 220), Coconut-Crusted Cod (page 241), Shredded Roast Beef (page 261), Citrus-Thyme Pot Roast (page 266)

POMEGRANATE AND ROCKET
SALAD WITH FENNEL

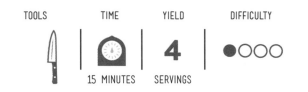

TOOLS	TIME	YIELD	DIFFICULTY
	15 MINUTES	4 SERVINGS	●○○○

140 g rocket leaves
1 small fennel bulb, thinly
   sliced
100 g pomegranate seeds
60 ml Blood Orange
   Vinaigrette (page 116)

1 Combine the rocket, fennel slices, and pomegranate seeds in a large bowl.

2 Toss with the vinaigrette and serve.

Variation: Substitute Apple Cider Vinaigrette (page 120) for a less sweet variation.

Storage: Keep dressing separate and toss through the salad right before serving.

Serving Suggestions: Coconut-Crusted Cod (page 241), Sear-Roasted Halibut (page 246), Citrus-Ginger Marinated Salmon (page 237)

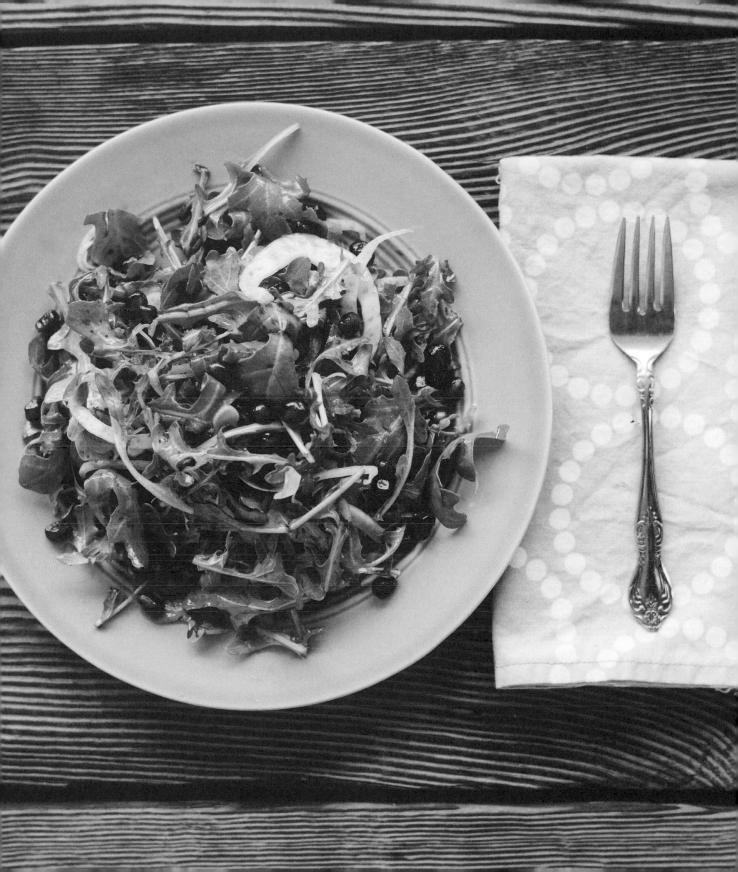

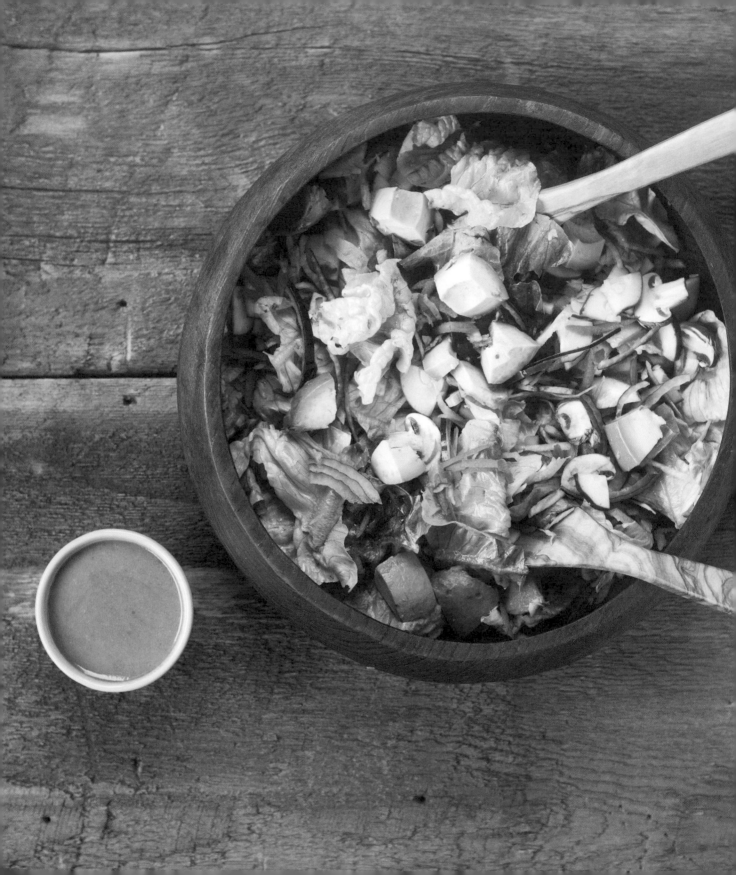

MARKET SALAD

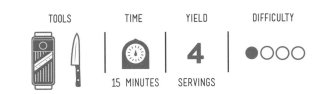

TOOLS | TIME | YIELD | DIFFICULTY

15 MINUTES | 4 SERVINGS | ●○○○

1 head soft lettuce, washed
 and leaves separated and torn
½ small red onion, thinly sliced
2 medium carrots, shredded
1 small beetroot, shredded
1 cucumber, thinly sliced
45 g button mushrooms,
 thinly sliced
230 ml of vinaigrette: Apple
 Cider (page 120), Ginger-Plum
 (page 120) or Blood Orange
 (page 116)
1 avocado, peeled, destoned
 and cubed

1 Combine the lettuce, onion, carrots, beetroot, cucumber and mushrooms in a large bowl.

2 Add your choice of vinaigrette to the salad and toss gently.

3 Top with fresh avocado and serve.

Storage: Keep dressing separate and toss (and add avocado) right before serving.

Serving Suggestions: Curried Chicken Salad (page 224), Mushroom-Stuffed Cornish Hens (page 223), Citrus-Ginger Marinated Salmon (page 237), Sole Fillet with Tarragon-Caper Sauce (page 245), Three-Herb Beef Patties (page 262)

CITRUS-SPINACH SALAD

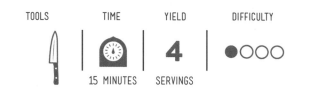

TOOLS TIME YIELD DIFFICULTY

15 MINUTES

4
SERVINGS

● ○ ○ ○

1 large bunch spinach, washed
   and stems trimmed
2 medium carrots, grated
10 kalamata olives, pitted
   and halved
½ cucumber, chopped
250 ml Citrus-Avocado
   Dressing (page 115)

1 Place the spinach, carrots, olives and cucumber in a large bowl.

2 Add the dressing to the salad and toss to combine.

Storage: Keep dressing separate and toss right before serving.

Serving Suggestions: Orange-Rosemary Duck (page 220), Mushroom-Stuffed Cornish Hens (page 223), Coconut-Crusted Cod (page 241), Sear-Roasted Halibut (page 246)

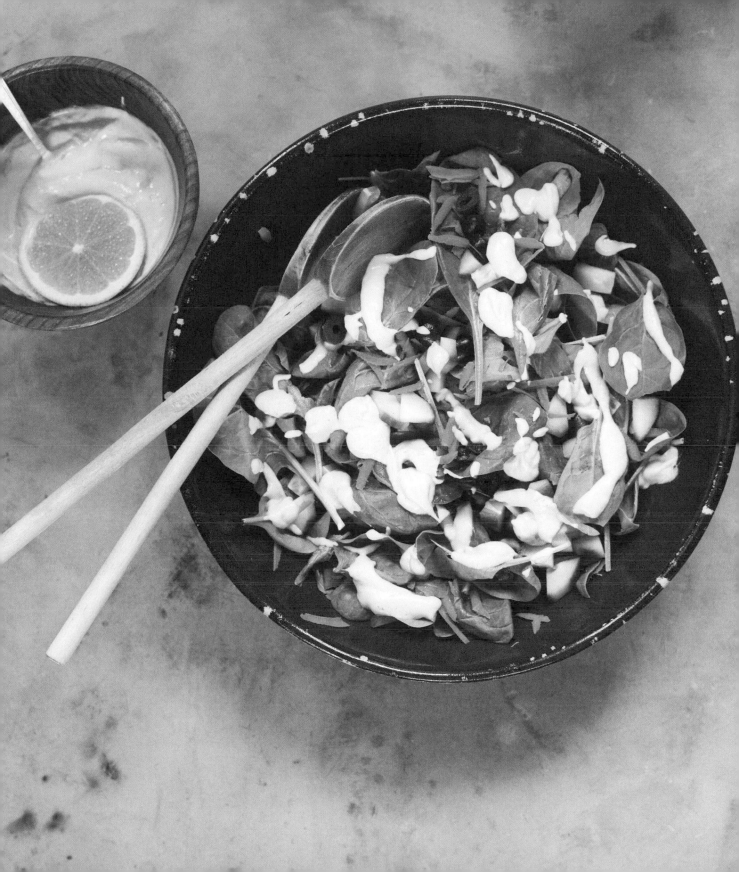

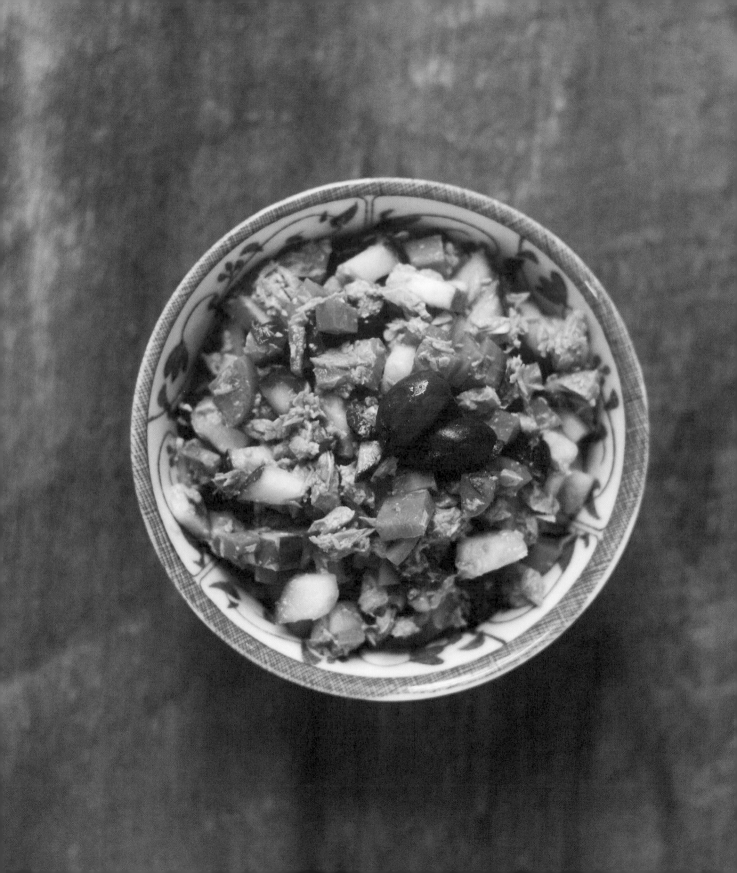

MEDITERRANEAN SALMON SALAD

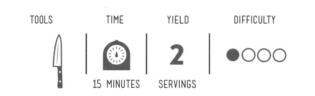

TOOLS | TIME | YIELD | DIFFICULTY

2

15 MINUTES | SERVINGS

●○○○

1 x 200 g tin BPA-free
   salmon, drained
2 medium carrots, finely
   chopped
½ cucumber, finely chopped
10 kalamata olives, pitted
   and halved
1 tablespoon chopped fresh
   flat-leaf parsley
3 tablespoons extra-virgin
   olive oil
Sea salt

1 Place the drained salmon in a small bowl and mash slightly to break it up.

2 Add the carrots, cucumber, olives, parsley, olive oil and salt, to taste. Toss gently to combine.

Storage: Keeps in the refrigerator for several days.

Serving Suggestions: Emerald Kale Salad (page 138), Cucumber-Mint Salad (page 141), Radish and Jicama Tabbouli (page 142), Market Salad (page 149)

CHICKEN CAESAR SALAD

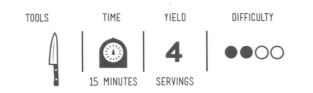

TOOLS	TIME	YIELD	DIFFICULTY
	15 MINUTES	4 SERVINGS	●●○○

1 large head romaine lettuce,
  chopped
1 bunch radishes, thinly sliced
900 g shredded chicken
  breast (page 212)
250 ml Caesar Salad Dressing,
  at room temperature
  (page 119)
1 avocado, peeled, destoned
  and cubed (optional)

1 Place the lettuce, radishes, shredded chicken and dressing in a large bowl and toss well to combine.

2 Add the avocado and serve immediately.

Storage: Keep dressing separate then toss through salad (and add avocado) right before serving.

Serving Suggestions: Rainbow Roasted Root Vegetables (page 188), Rosemary-Roasted Carrots and Parsnips (page 203), Roasted Mixed Vegetables (page 199)

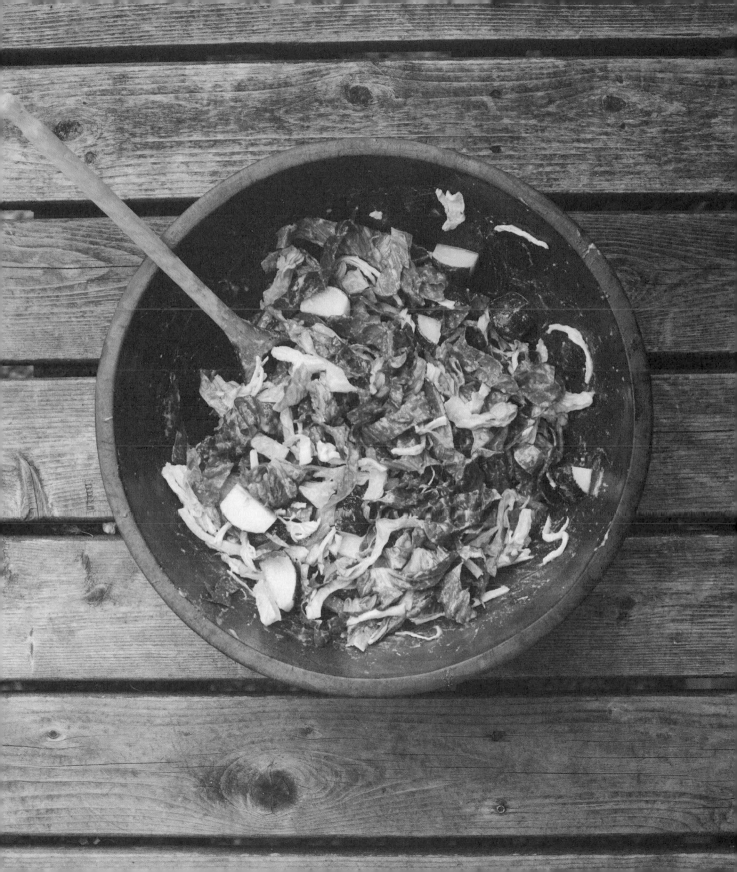

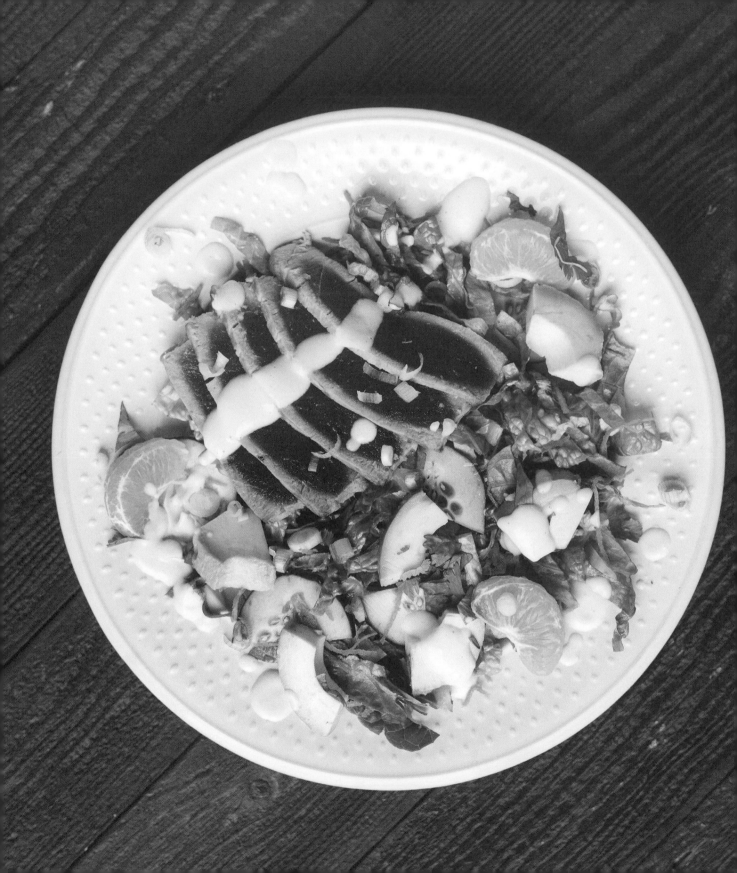

SEARED TUNA SALAD WITH CITRUS-AVOCADO DRESSING

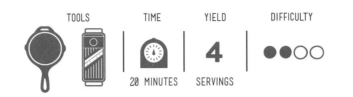

TOOLS

TIME
20 MINUTES

YIELD
4 SERVINGS

DIFFICULTY
●●○○

4 x 175 g tuna steaks, at room temperature

¼ teaspoon sea salt

1 tablespoon coconut oil

1 large head romaine lettuce, shredded

1 carrot, grated

1 cucumber, halved and sliced thinly

1 avocado, peeled, destoned and cubed

1 tangerine, sectioned

250 ml Citrus-Avocado Dressing (page 115)

1 Salt the tuna on both sides.

2 Heat the coconut oil in a large frying pan on medium–high heat until lightly smoking.

3 Sear the tuna for about 1½ minutes per side (for medium rare), or until it reaches your desired doneness. Remove from heat, slice thinly, and set aside.

4 Place the lettuce, grated carrot and cucumber in a bowl and toss to combine.

5 Divide the lettuce mixture between several plates; add portions of seared tuna, avocado cubes and tangerine segments. Serve with dressing poured over the top.

Storage: Serve this salad the day you make it.

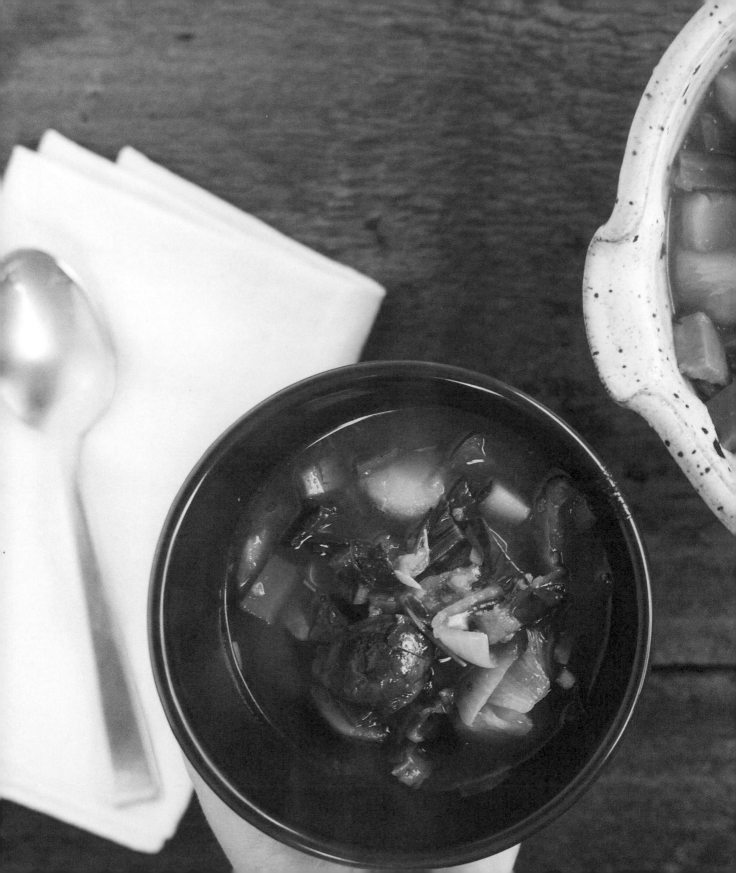

SOUPS + STEWS

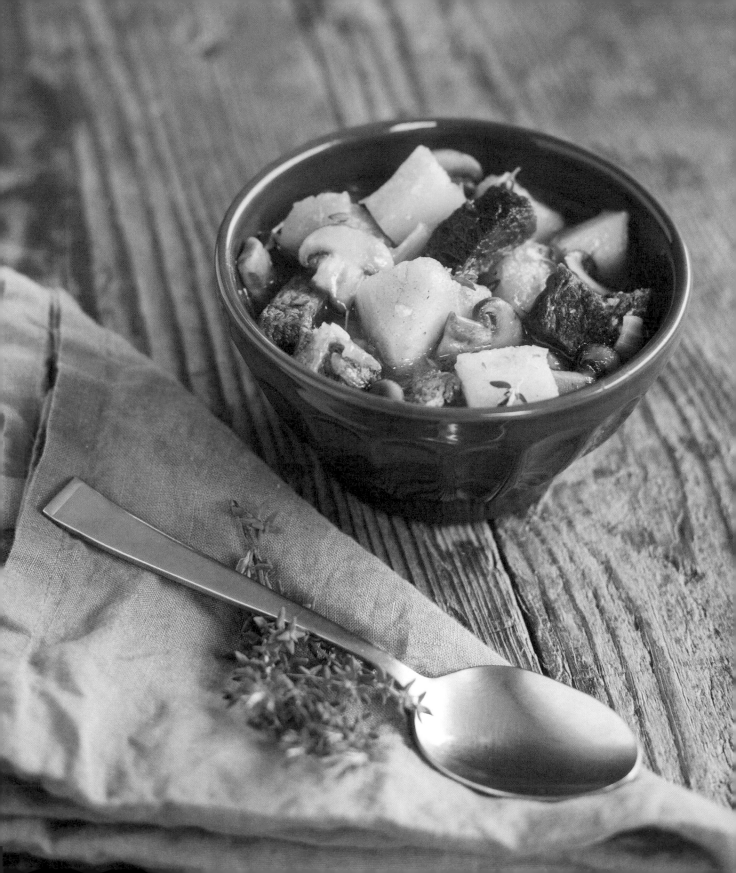

BEEF-BUTTERNUT STEW WITH PEAR AND THYME

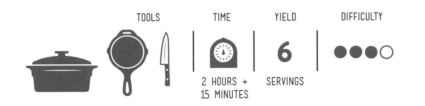

TOOLS	TIME	YIELD	DIFFICULTY
	2 HOURS + 15 MINUTES	**6** SERVINGS	●●●○

2 tablespoons solid cooking fat

900 g–1.3 kg free-range stewing beef, cut into 4 cm cubes

1 large onion, chopped

5 cm piece ginger, peeled and minced

5 cloves garlic, minced

500 ml Bone Broth (page 34)

1 bay leaf

1 small butternut squash, peeled and cubed

½ teaspoon ground cinnamon

½ teaspoon sea salt

2 firm pears, peeled and chopped

90 g sliced mushrooms, for garnish

1 tablespoon chopped fresh thyme, for garnish

1 Heat 1 tablespoon of the cooking fat in a heavy-bottomed pot on medium–high heat.

2 When the fat has melted and the pan is hot, brown the meat in batches. Remove from the pot, and turn the heat down to medium.

3 Add the onion and cook for about 5 minutes, stirring, until it begins to soften. Add the ginger and garlic, and cook for another couple of minutes, being careful to stir so the onion doesn't burn.

4 Return the meat to the pot, add the bone broth and bay leaf, and bring to a boil. Immediately turn down to a bare simmer. Cover tightly and cook for 45 minutes.

5 Add the butternut squash, cinnamon and salt and continue to simmer, covered, for another 15 minutes.

6 Add the pears and simmer for another 30 minutes, or until the meat and squash are both tender.

7 In a small frying pan, heat the rest of the cooking fat on medium–high heat and sauté the mushrooms for about 5 minutes, or until they are soft and have browned slightly.

8 Remove the bay leaf. Serve the stew in bowls, garnished with the sautéed mushrooms and a sprinkle of fresh thyme.

Storage: Keeps well in the refrigerator for several days; also freezes well.

BEETROOT-FENNEL SOUP

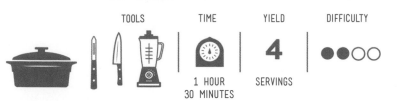

TOOLS | TIME | YIELD | DIFFICULTY

1 HOUR 30 MINUTES | 4 SERVINGS | ●●○○

2 tablespoons solid cooking fat
1 large fennel bulb, ends removed and fronds reserved, bulb thinly sliced
2 cloves garlic, minced
2.5 cm piece ginger, peeled and minced
750 ml Bone Broth (page 34)
900 g beetroot, peeled and cut into 4 cm chunks
1 bay leaf
1 teaspoon sea salt
½ lemon, juiced (about 1 tablespoon)

1 In a heavy-bottomed pot, melt the cooking fat on medium heat. When the pan is hot, sauté the sliced fennel for about 10 minutes, or until it softens. Add the garlic and ginger to the pot and cook for a few more minutes, stirring.

2 Add the broth, beetroot, bay leaf and salt. Bring to a boil, cover, then turn down to a simmer. Cook for 1 hour and 15 minutes, or until the beetroot is very tender.

3 Remove the bay leaf. Carefully transfer the soup to a high-powered blender or food processor. Blend until desired consistency is reached, adding more broth if needed. Serve warm, with a squeeze of lemon juice and fennel fronds to garnish.

Storage: Keeps well in the refrigerator for several days; also freezes well.

CARROT-GINGER SOUP

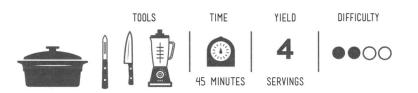

TOOLS | TIME | YIELD | DIFFICULTY

45 MINUTES | 4 SERVINGS | ●●○○

2 tablespoons solid cooking fat
1 small onion, chopped
5 cm piece of ginger, peeled and minced
3 cloves garlic, minced
900 g carrots (about 6 medium), chopped
1 tablespoon apple cider vinegar
1 litre Bone Broth (page 34)
1 bay leaf
½ teaspoon ground cinnamon
1½ teaspoons sea salt
1 tablespoon minced chives, for garnish

1 Heat the cooking fat over medium heat in a heavy-bottomed pot until melted. Add the onion, and cook for about 5 minutes, stirring, until it begins to soften. Add the ginger and garlic and cook for a couple more minutes, stirring to ensure nothing burns. Add the carrots and cook for another 10 minutes, stirring often.

2 Add the vinegar, bone broth, bay leaf, cinnamon and salt to the pot. Bring to a boil, turn down to a gentle simmer and cover tightly with a lid. Cook for 20 minutes, or until carrots are very soft.

3 Turn off the heat, remove the bay leaf and carefully transfer the soup to a high-powered blender or food processor. Purée until the soup reaches your desired thickness, adding more broth if needed. Serve with a sprinkle of chives for garnish.

Storage: Keeps well in the refrigerator for several days; also freezes well.

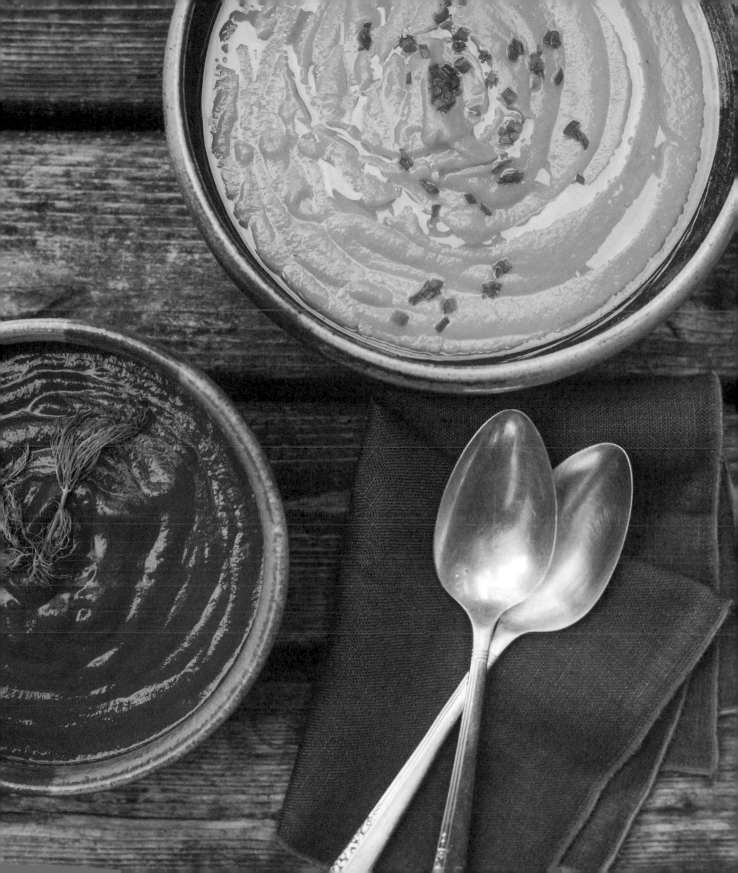

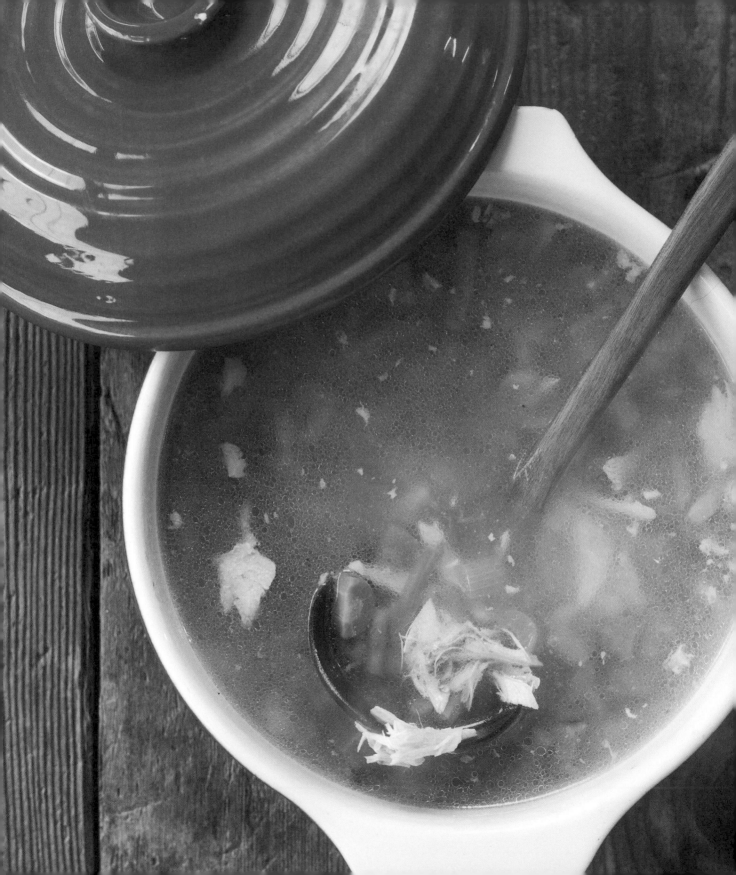

CLASSIC CHICKEN SOUP

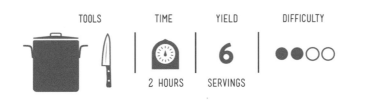

TOOLS | TIME | YIELD | DIFFICULTY
2 HOURS | 6 SERVINGS | ●●○○

1 x 1.8–2.25 kg chicken
1 large onion, chopped
1 bay leaf
2 cloves garlic
1 tablespoon sea salt, plus more
  as needed
6 large carrots, chopped
6 celery stalks, chopped
900 g green beans, chopped

1 Begin by cleaning the chicken (rinse it under cold water and remove any loose bits of fat and other tissue). Place it in a large stockpot. If it doesn't fit, you will have to cut it into quarters.

2 Add the onion, bay leaf, garlic and salt. Fill the pot with cold water until the chicken is just covered. Bring to a boil, then cover tightly and lower the heat to a bare simmer. Cook this way until the meat is tender and falling off the bone, about 1 to 2 hours—the lower the simmer, the more tender your chicken will be. Skim the surface of the broth to remove any scum that may appear during cooking.

3 Remove the chicken from the pot and set it aside. Pour the vegetables and broth through a sieve, being careful to save the broth! Discard the vegetables and the bay leaf.

4 Add the broth back to the pot along with the carrots, celery, and green beans. Bring to a boil, then lower the heat. Cover and cook at a simmer for about 20 minutes, or until the vegetables are tender.

5 While the vegetables are cooking, remove the meat from the chicken carcass and set it aside in a bowl.

6 When the veggies are tender, add the meat back to the soup and simmer for another 20 minutes. Add more salt to taste and serve.

Storage: Keeps well in the refrigerator for several days; also freezes well.

COLD AVOCADO-CUCUMBER SOUP

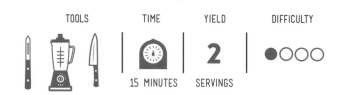

TOOLS	TIME	YIELD	DIFFICULTY

15 MINUTES   2 SERVINGS   ●○○○

1 avocado

2 large cucumbers, chopped

185 ml filtered water

60 ml extra-virgin olive oil,
plus more for serving

2 tablespoons chopped
fresh mint

2.5 cm piece ginger, peeled
and minced

1 clove garlic

½ lemon, juiced
(about 1 tablespoon)

½ tablespoon apple cider
vinegar

½ teaspoon sea salt

Fresh mint or coriander leaves,
for garnish

Olive oil, for drizzling

1 Make sure all ingredients are well chilled when you begin this recipe so that the finished soup will be cold when served.

3 Cut the avocado in half, then destone and peel it. Cut one of the halves into slices and set them aside. Place the other half and all of the remaining ingredients (except the olive oil and herbs for garnish) in a high-powered blender and blend on high until perfectly smooth.

3 Serve immediately, topped with the avocado slices, a few mint or coriander leaves and a drizzle of olive oil.

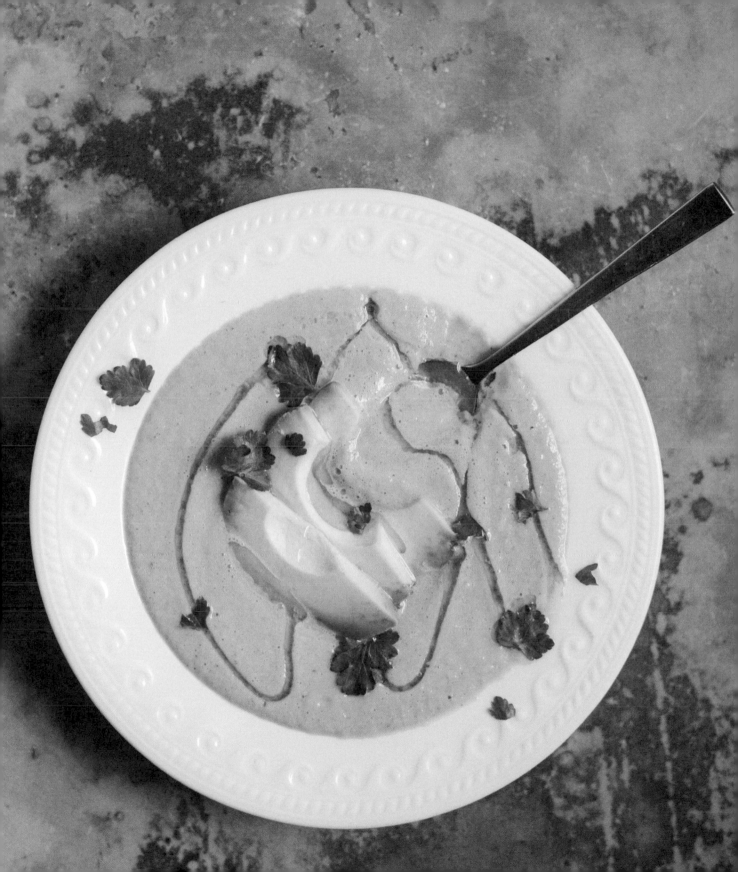

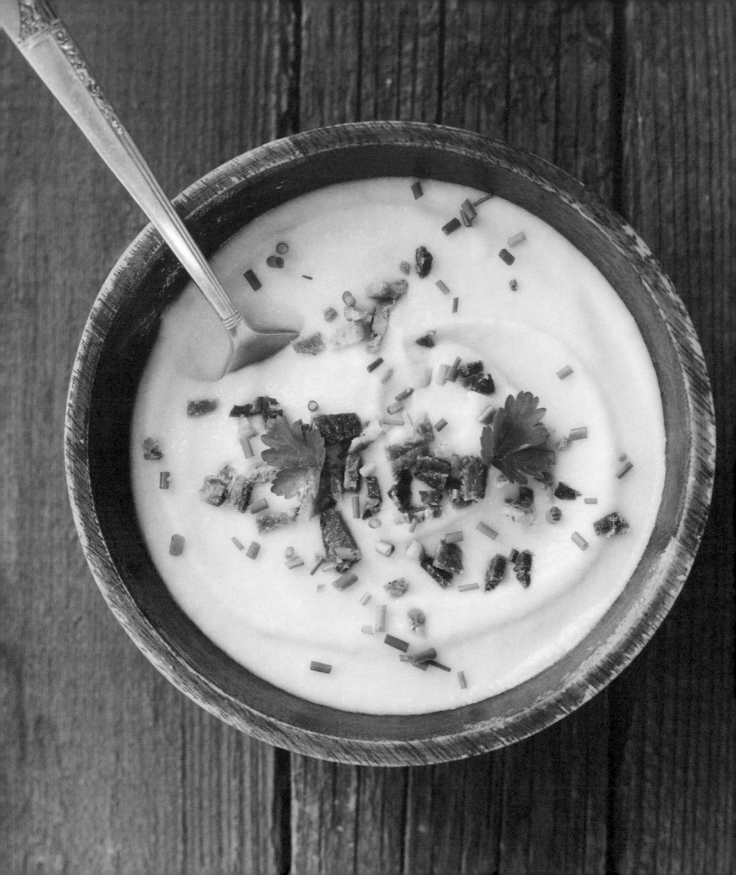

CREAMY CELERIAC AND LEEK SOUP

TOOLS   TIME   YIELD   DIFFICULTY

4

45 MINUTES   SERVINGS

4 rashers sugar-free bacon

2 leeks, washed, ends removed,
and sliced thinly

3 cloves garlic, minced

2.5 cm piece ginger, peeled
and minced

1 litre Bone Broth (page 34)

900 g celeriac, peeled and
cut into 4 cm chunks

1 tablespoon apple cider vinegar

½ teaspoon sea salt

1 bay leaf

A few sprigs of fresh flat-leaf
parsley, for garnish

1 Add the bacon to a heavy-bottomed pot over medium heat. Cook until crispy, flipping as needed. Remove the bacon to cool, leaving the fat in the bottom of the pan.

2 Add the leeks and cook for 5 minutes, stirring. Add the garlic and ginger and cook, stirring, for another couple of minutes.

3 Add the broth, celeriac, vinegar, salt and bay leaf and bring to a boil. Turn down to a simmer, cover, and cook for 15 minutes, or until celeriac is soft.

4 While the soup is cooking, crumble the bacon into small bits.

5 Remove the bay leaf, transfer the soup to a blender and process until desired consistency is reached, adding more broth if needed.

6 Serve garnished with parsley and crumbled bacon on top.

Storage: Keeps well in the refrigerator for several days; also freezes well.

WINTER SQUASH SOUP

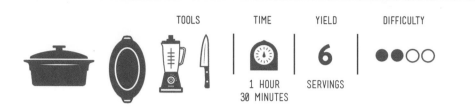

TOOLS   TIME   YIELD   DIFFICULTY

6

1 HOUR   SERVINGS
30 MINUTES

●●○○

1.8 kg kabocha squash, halved, seeds removed

3 tablespoons solid cooking fat

1 onion, chopped

4 cloves garlic, minced

500 ml Bone Broth (page 34), plus more as needed

1 teaspoon sea salt

1 teaspoon ground cinnamon

Sliced avocado, for garnish

Chopped fresh flat-leaf parsley, for garnish

1 Preheat the oven to 200°C.

2 Place the squash cut-side up in a baking dish. Spread 2 tablespoons of the cooking fat all over the flesh of the squash and on the bottom of the pan. Roast for 1 hour, or until completely tender.

3 While the squash is roasting, heat the remaining tablespoon of the cooking fat in a large, heavy-bottomed pot. Cook the onion for about 10 minutes, stirring, and then add the garlic for a couple of minutes, stirring. Set aside.

4 Remove the squash from the oven and allow it to cool enough to handle. Scoop out the flesh and blend in batches with the onion mixture, bone broth, salt, and cinnamon. If the soup is too thick, add more broth or water, 60 ml at a time, until desired consistency is reached.

5 Pour the purée back into the large pot and reheat, adding salt to taste. Serve with slices of avocado and parsley for garnish.

Variation: Feel free to use any other type of hard winter squash for this recipe—butternut, acorn, and pumpkin all work well.

Storage: Keeps well in the refrigerator for several days; also freezes well (both without the avocado).

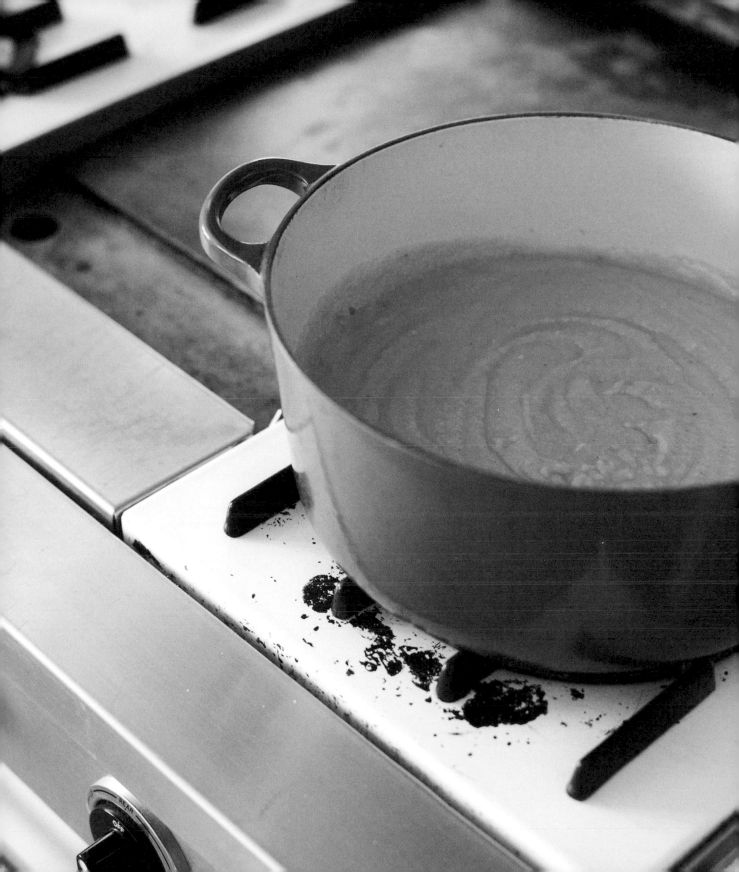

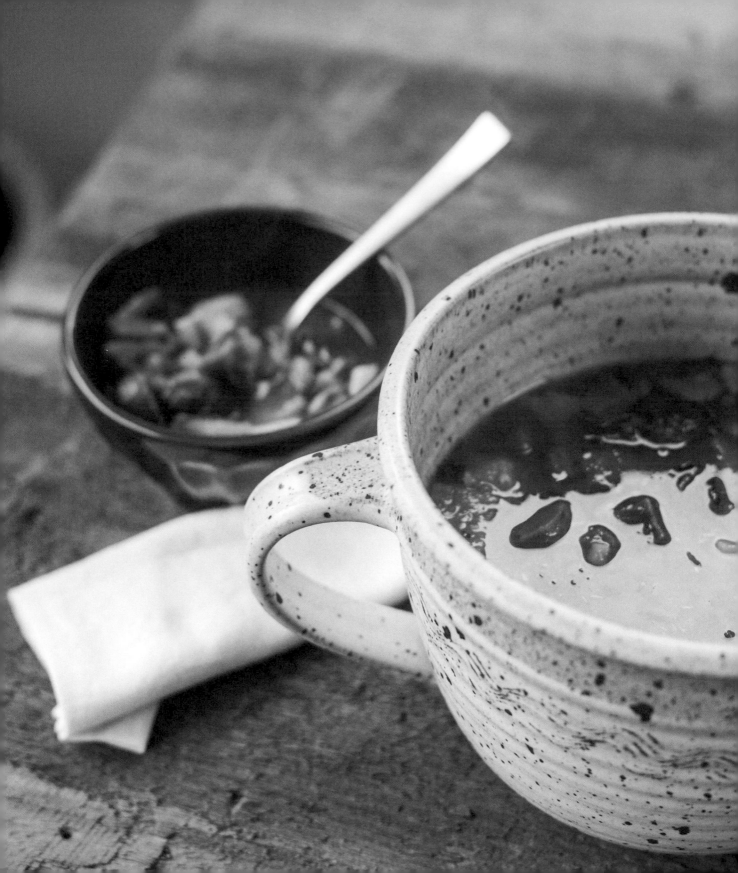

HEARTY VEGETABLE SOUP

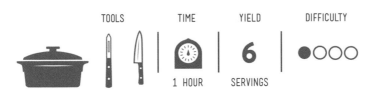

TOOLS	TIME	YIELD	DIFFICULTY
	1 HOUR	**6** SERVINGS	●○○○

1 tablespoon solid cooking fat

1 large onion, chopped

3 cloves garlic, minced

2.5 cm piece ginger, peeled and
   minced

4 carrots, cut into 4 cm chunks

2 parsnips, cut into 4 cm chunks

1 large sweet potato, peeled
   and cut into 4 cm chunks

90 g crimini mushrooms, halved

1 tablespoon chopped rosemary

1 tablespoon chopped thyme

1 tablespoon apple cider vinegar

2 litres Bone Broth (page 34)

1 bay leaf

1 teaspoon sea salt

1 bunch chard, stems removed,
   leaves chopped

1 Heat the cooking fat in a heavy-bottomed pot over medium–high heat. Add the onion and cook, stirring, for 5 minutes. Add the garlic and ginger; cook for another couple of minutes, stirring. Add the carrots, parsnips, sweet potato, mushrooms, rosemary and thyme, and sauté for another 5 minutes, or until the outsides of the vegetables are lightly browned.

2 Add the vinegar, bone broth, bay leaf, and salt. Bring to a boil, then reduce the heat, cover, and let the soup simmer gently. Cook for about 20 minutes, or until the vegetables are tender.

3 Add the chard during the last couple minutes of cooking, and let the pieces soften in the warm broth. Check to see that the broth is salty enough; add more salt if needed. Remove the bay leaf before serving.

Variation: Feel free to switch up the root vegetables in this recipe; turnip and swede are nice choices if they are available. You can also use kale or spring greens instead of the chard.

Storage: Keeps well in the refrigerator for several days; also freezes well.

MOROCCAN LAMB STEW

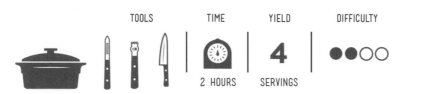

TOOLS · TIME — 2 HOURS · YIELD — 4 SERVINGS · DIFFICULTY ●●○○

½ teaspoon ground cinnamon

1 teaspoon sea salt

900 g stewing lamb

2 tablespoons solid cooking fat

1 onion, chopped

4 cloves garlic, minced

5 cm piece ginger, peeled and minced

2 tablespoons minced fresh rosemary

1 tablespoon apple cider vinegar

125 ml Bone Broth (page 34)

125 ml filtered water

620 g chopped carrots

5 dates, pitted and minced

2 small blood oranges, zested and juiced (reserve 1 teaspoon zest)

A small handful chopped coriander, for garnish

1 In a small bowl, combine the cinnamon and sea salt and use it to coat the stewing meat.

2 Heat the fat in a heavy-bottomed pot on medium heat. When the fat has melted and the pan is hot, brown the meat in batches. Remove the meat from the pot and set aside. Add the onion and cook for 5 minutes, stirring. Next add the garlic, ginger, and rosemary, and cook for another couple of minutes, until fragrant.

3 Add the vinegar, bone broth, water, carrots, dates and blood-orange juice (you should have about 80 ml) to the pot with the lamb; bring to a boil. Turn down to a bare simmer, cover, and cook for about 1½ hours, until the lamb and veggies are all tender.

4 Stir in the orange zest. Serve garnished with coriander.

Variation: Feel free to use any other type of red meat in this recipe if you do not have lamb available to you. Also, regular oranges will work well if you cannot find blood oranges.

Storage: Keeps well in the refrigerator for several days; also freezes well.

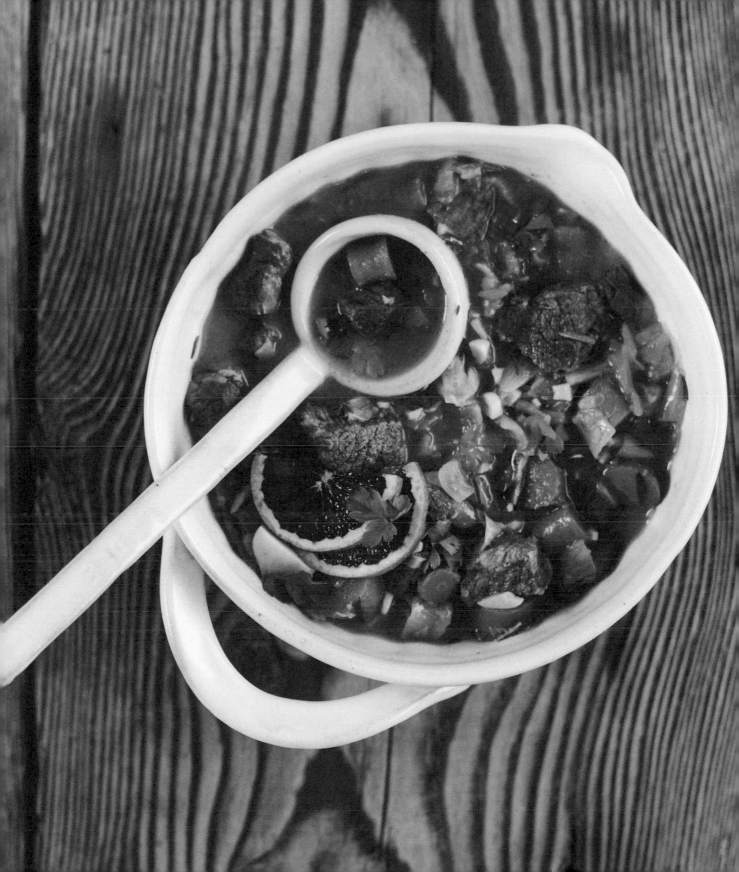

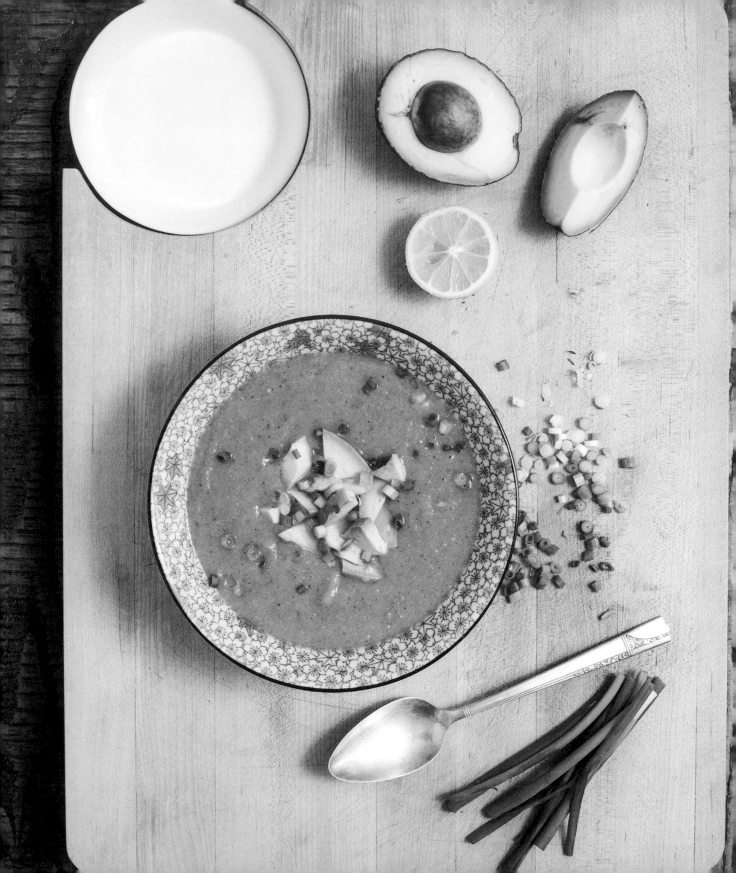

UNDER THE WEATHER SOUP

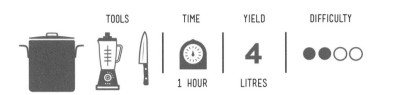

TOOLS	TIME	YIELD	DIFFICULTY
	1 HOUR	**4** LITRES	●●○○

2 litres Bone Broth (page 34)

950 ml filtered water

3 medium sweet potatoes, peeled and roughly chopped

1 teaspoon sea salt

450 g green beans, roughly chopped

2 courgettes (zucchini), roughly chopped

1 bunch leafy greens (like kale or chard), stems removed and leaves roughly chopped

4 cloves garlic, peeled and chopped

5 cm piece ginger, peeled and chopped

Juice of 1 lemon (about 2 tablespoons), for serving

1 avocado, peeled, destoned and thinly sliced, for garnish

1 Place the bone broth, water, sweet potatoes and salt in a large stockpot and bring to a boil. Turn down to a simmer and cook for 20 to 30 minutes, or until the sweet potatoes are tender.

2 Turn off the heat and add the green beans, courgette and leafy greens. Cover and let the soup sit for a few minutes, so that the vegetables soften a little but don't cook. Add the garlic and ginger.

3 Blend the soup in batches and transfer it to another large pot. Reheat gently.

4 Serve with additional salt as needed, a squeeze of lemon juice and avocado slices.

Variation: Use winter squash instead of sweet potatoes. You can also replace the filtered water with more bone broth for a super-healing variation.

Storage: Keeps well in the refrigerator for several days; also freezes well.

CURRIED CHICKEN AND VEGETABLE SOUP

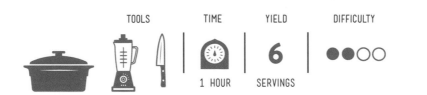

TOOLS | TIME 1 HOUR | YIELD 6 SERVINGS | DIFFICULTY ●●○○

1 tablespoon solid cooking fat

1 onion, chopped

4 cloves garlic, minced

4 cm piece ginger, peeled and minced

1 litre Bone Broth (page 34)

900 g celeriac, peeled and cut into 5 cm chunks

1 carrot, cut into thin rounds

1 tablespoon ground turmeric

1 teaspoon sea salt

500 ml Creamy Coconut Milk (page 46)

90 g thinly sliced mushrooms,

900 g shredded chicken breast meat (page 212)

1 lime, juiced (about ½ tablespoon)

A small handful chopped coriander, for garnish

1 Heat the cooking fat in the bottom of a heavy-bottomed pot on medium. When the fat has melted and the pan is hot, add the onion and cook, stirring, for 5 minutes. Add the garlic and ginger, and cook for another couple of minutes, stirring.

2 Add the bone broth, celeriac, carrot, turmeric and salt to the pot. Bring to a boil, then reduce the heat to low and simmer, covered, for 20 minutes.

3 Remove 500 ml of the soup and purée in a blender. Return the purée to the pot; add the mushrooms and shredded chicken. Simmer for another 10 minutes.

4 Serve each bowl with a squeeze of lime and a sprinkle of fresh coriander.

Storage: Keeps well in the refrigerator for several days; also freezes well.

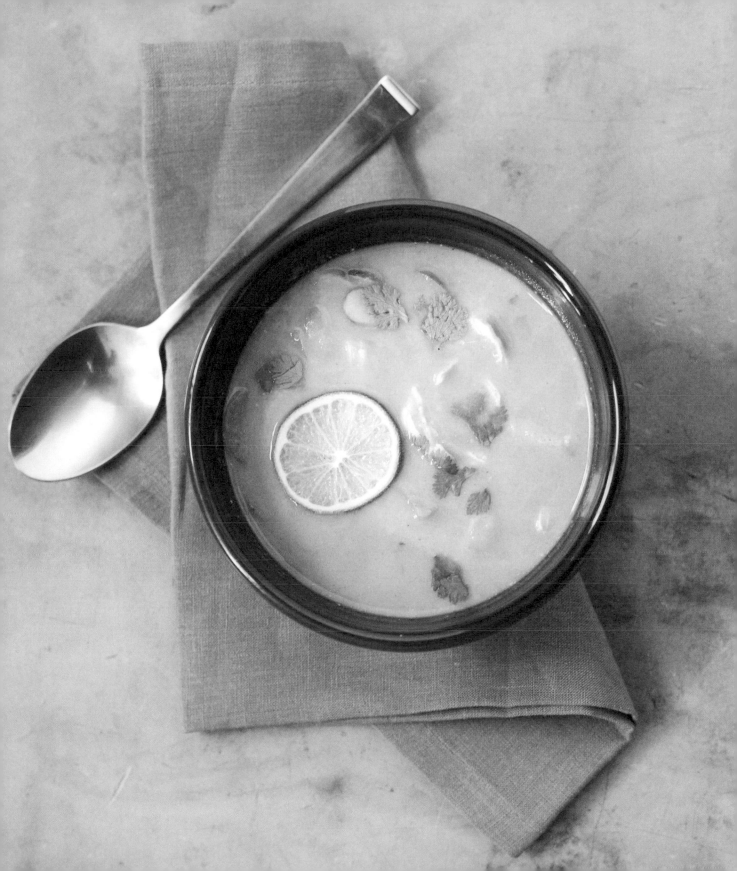

VEGETABLES

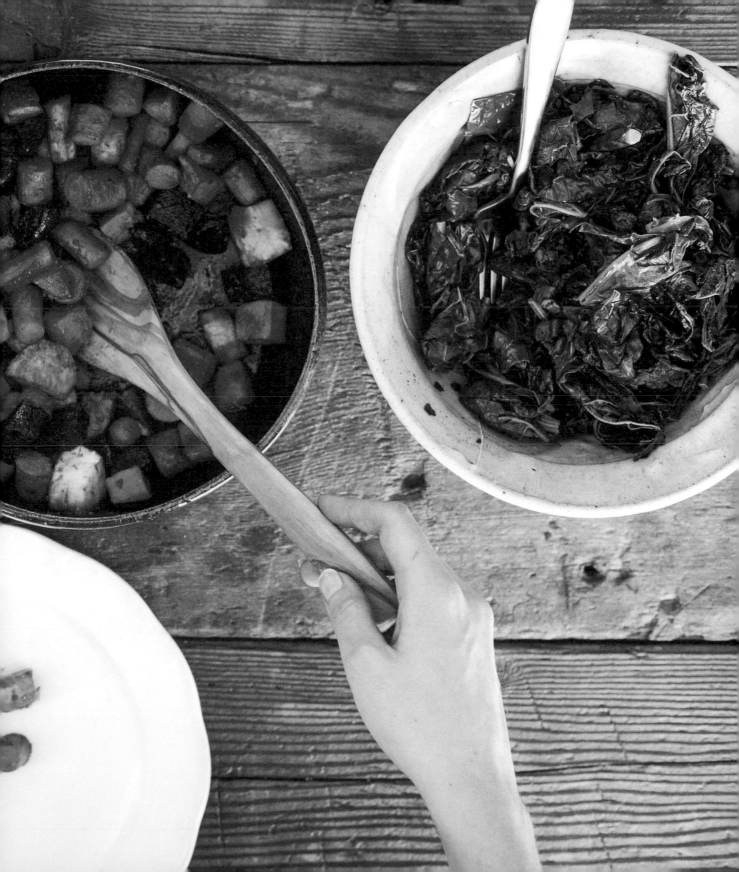

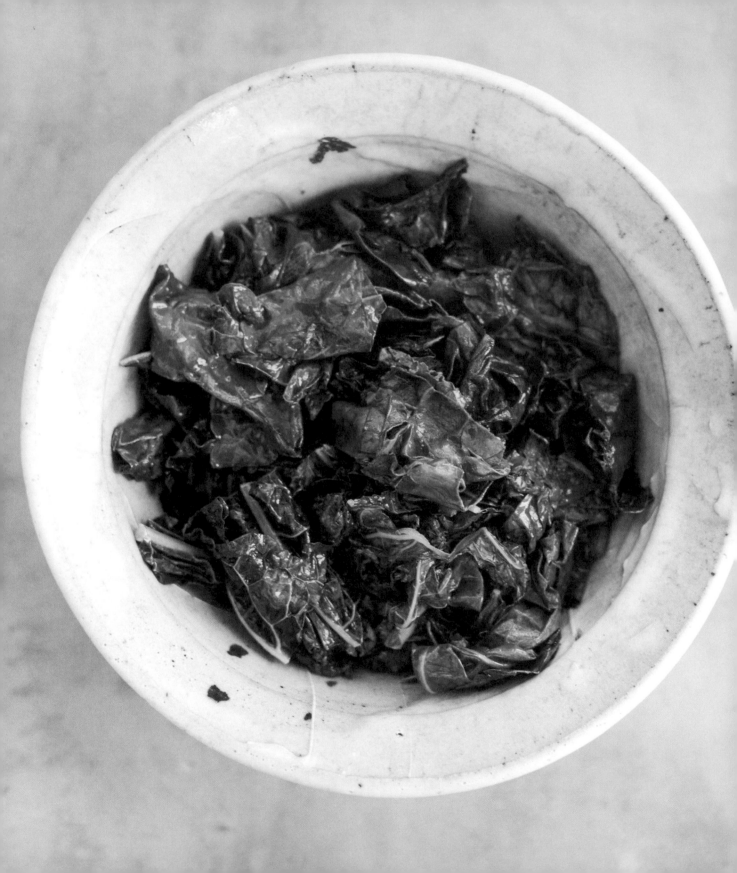

SAUTÉED MARKET GREENS

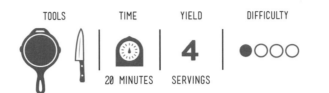

TOOLS | TIME | YIELD | DIFFICULTY

20 MINUTES | 4 SERVINGS | ●○○○

2 large bunches kale, chard or spring greens, stems removed and leaves roughly chopped

2 tablespoons solid cooking fat

1 teaspoon sea salt

1 Wash and dry the greens thoroughly, making sure they are not too wet before cooking.

2 Heat the cooking fat in a large frying pan on medium heat. When the fat has melted and the pan is hot, add the greens in batches, stirring as they cook. It's OK if they don't all fit in the pan at once—just keep adding more of the raw pieces as the others cook down. Add the salt and cook for about 15 minutes, stirring, or until tender. Serve warm.

Variation: Feel free to use any varieties of large-leafed brassica vegetables (also known as cruciferous vegetables, cabbages, or mustards) for this recipe.

Storage: Keeps in the refrigerator for several days.

Serving Suggestions: Coconut-Basil Pesto (page 124), Roasted Mixed Vegetables (page 199), Cinnamon-Scented Butternut Squash (page 184), Lemon-Garlic Marinated Chicken (page 219), Sage-Braised Chicken Legs (page 228), Orange Duck (page 220), Sear-Roasted Halibut (page 246), Braised Lamb Shanks (page 273), Rosemary Shredded Beef (page 278)

CINNAMON-SCENTED BUTTERNUT SQUASH

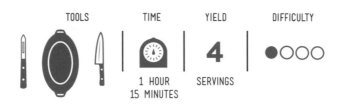

TOOLS	TIME	YIELD	DIFFICULTY
	1 HOUR 15 MINUTES	4 SERVINGS	●○○○

1.3 kg butternut squash, peeled, seeds removed, and cut into 4 cm cubes

2 tablespoons solid cooking fat, melted

¼ teaspoon ground cinnamon

⅛ teaspoon ground ginger

¼ teaspoon sea salt

1 Preheat the oven to 200°C.

2 Place the butternut squash in a large bowl and combine with the cooking fat, cinnamon, ginger and salt, stirring to coat evenly.

3 Place in a baking dish and cook for 1 hour, or until completely tender, making sure to stir every 20 minutes or so. Serve warm.

Variation: Feel free to use any type of winter squash for this recipe—pumpkin, acorn and kabocha all work well.

Storage: Keeps in the refrigerator for several days.

Serving Suggestions: Sautéed Market Greens (page 183), Rosemary Grilled Asparagus (page 195), Chicken and Pesto Sauté (page 216), Lemon-Garlic Marinated Chicken (page 219), Herbed Roast Chicken (page 227)

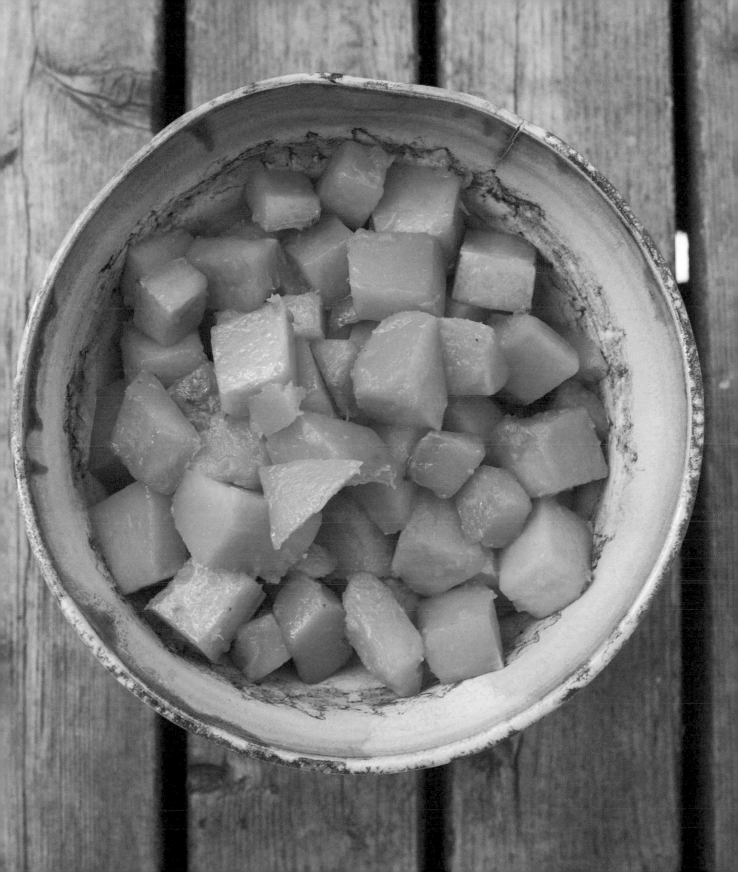

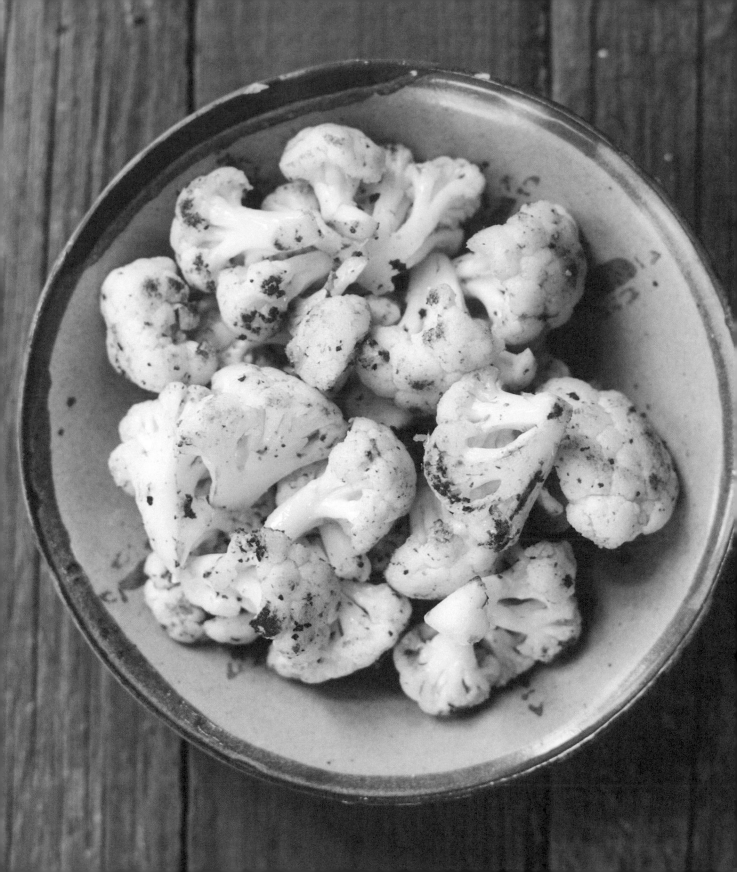

CURRIED CAULIFLOWER

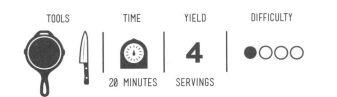

TOOLS | TIME | YIELD | DIFFICULTY

20 MINUTES | **4** SERVINGS | ●○○○

2 tablespoons solid cooking fat

1 large head cauliflower, chopped into 2.5 cm pieces

½ teaspoon ground turmeric

½ teaspoon ground ginger

¼ teaspoon sea salt

1 tablespoon coconut aminos (optional)

1 Heat the fat in a wok or large frying pan on medium heat.

2 When the fat has melted and the pan is hot, add the cauliflower and sprinkle with the turmeric, ginger and salt, stirring to combine. Cover and cook for 10 minutes or until the cauliflower is just tender, stirring a couple of times.

3 Add the coconut aminos and cook for another minute.

Variation: Sauté some minced shallots and garlic before adding the cauliflower.

Storage: Keeps in the refrigerator for several days.

Serving Suggestions: Asian-Marinated Grilled Chicken (page 219), Citrus-Ginger Marinated Salmon (page 237), Shrimp and Green Bean Stir-Fry (page 249), Garlic Beef and Broccoli (page 270)

RAINBOW ROASTED ROOT VEGETABLES

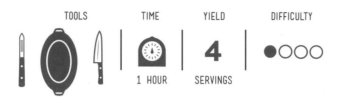

TOOLS	TIME	YIELD	DIFFICULTY
	1 HOUR	4 SERVINGS	●○○○

5 medium carrots, cut into 2.5 cm pieces

3 medium beetroots, peeled and cut into 2.5 cm pieces

3 medium parsnips, peeled and cut into 2.5 cm pieces

1 small swede, peeled and cut into 2.5 cm pieces

3 tablespoons solid cooking fat, melted

½ teaspoon sea salt

1 Preheat the oven to 200°C.

2 Combine the carrots, beetroots, parsnips and swede in a bowl and coat with the cooking fat and salt.

3 Transfer to a baking dish and bake until soft and browned on the outside (about 1 hour). Make sure to stir a couple of times while cooking. Serve warm.

Note: Feel free to use your own mixture of root vegetables for this recipe, not just the ones called for. Sweet potato, celeriac and turnip make lovely additions to, or substitutions for, any of the above.

Storage: Keeps in the refrigerator for several days.

Serving Suggestions: Brussels Sprouts with Crispy Bacon (page 191), Sautéed Market Greens (page 183), Seared Broccolini and Basil-Pesto (page 204), Herbed Roast Chicken (page 227), Mushroom-Stuffed Cornish Hens (page 223), Citrus-Ginger Marinated Salmon (page 237), Herb Stuffed Trout (page 253), Cranberry-Braised Beef Short Ribs (page 258)

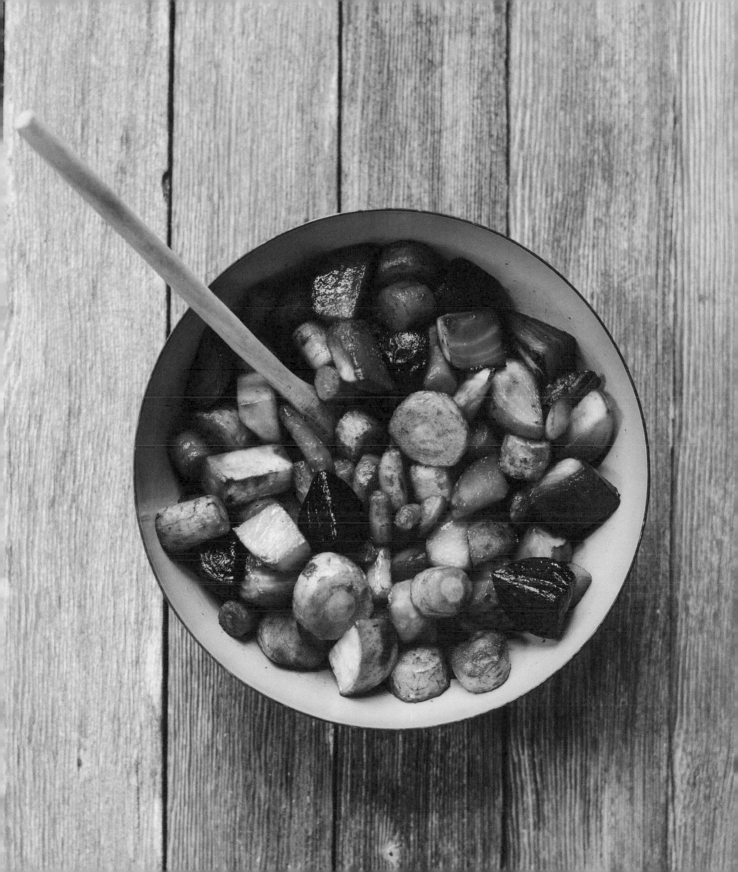

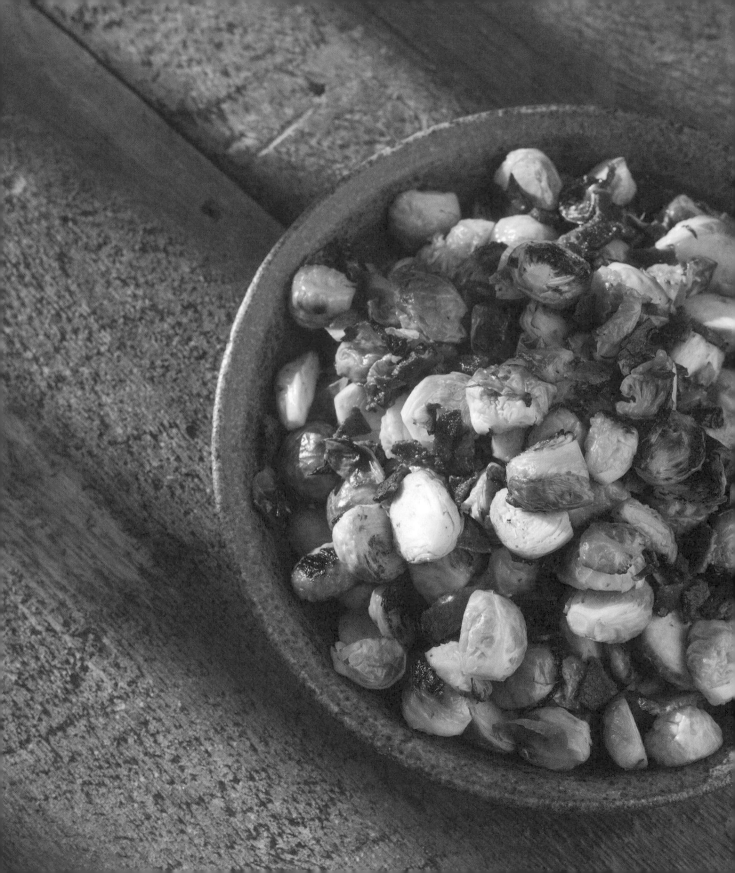

BRUSSELS SPROUTS
WITH CRISPY BACON

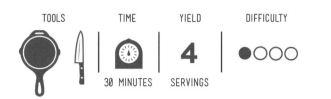

TOOLS	TIME	YIELD	DIFFICULTY
	30 MINUTES	4 SERVINGS	●○○○

680 g brussels sprouts
6 rashers sugar-free bacon
Sea salt

1 Wash brussels sprouts, cut the stem ends off, slice in half and set aside.

2 Cook bacon in a frying pan over medium heat until crispy, turning as necessary. Remove and set bacon aside to cool, leaving the fat in the pan.

3 Sauté brussels sprouts for about 15 minutes, or until browned on the outside and cooked through.

4 When the bacon has cooled, chop into small bits. Combine with the brussels sprouts and serve warm.

Variation: Substitute any green vegetable for the brussels sprouts, making sure to adjust the cooking time accordingly. Broccoli, kale, chard or spring greens are all good options.

Storage: Keeps well in the refrigerator for several days, although the bacon loses its crispness.

Serving Suggestions: Garlic-Sage Chicken Patties (page 211), Lemon-Garlic Marinated Chicken (page 219), Cranberry-Braised Beef Short Ribs (page 258), Lamb Chops with Rosemary-Plum Sauce (page 281)

MASHED SWEET POTATOES

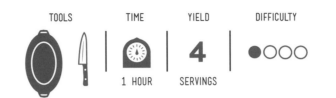

TOOLS | TIME | YIELD | DIFFICULTY

1 HOUR | 4 SERVINGS | ●○○○

680 g sweet potatoes (about 2 large), peeled and cubed

1 tablespoon solid cooking fat, melted, plus more as needed

¼ teaspoon sea salt

1 Preheat the oven to 200°C.

2 Combine the sweet potato, cooking fat and salt in a bowl, making sure to coat evenly.

3 Place in a baking dish and cook for 40 minutes or until soft, stirring a couple of times while cooking.

4 Remove from the oven, place in a bowl and mash with a potato masher, adding more fat until desired consistency is reached. Serve warm.

Variation: Feel free to use winter squash instead of sweet potato for this recipe.

Storage: Keeps in the refrigerator for several days.

Serving Suggestions: Sautéed Market Greens (page 183), Rosemary Grilled Asparagus (page 195), Herbed Roast Chicken (page 227), Sage-Braised Chicken Legs (page 228), Mushroom Stuffed Cornish Hens (page 223), Herb-Stuffed Whole Trout (page 253), Citrus-Thyme Pot Roast (page 266)

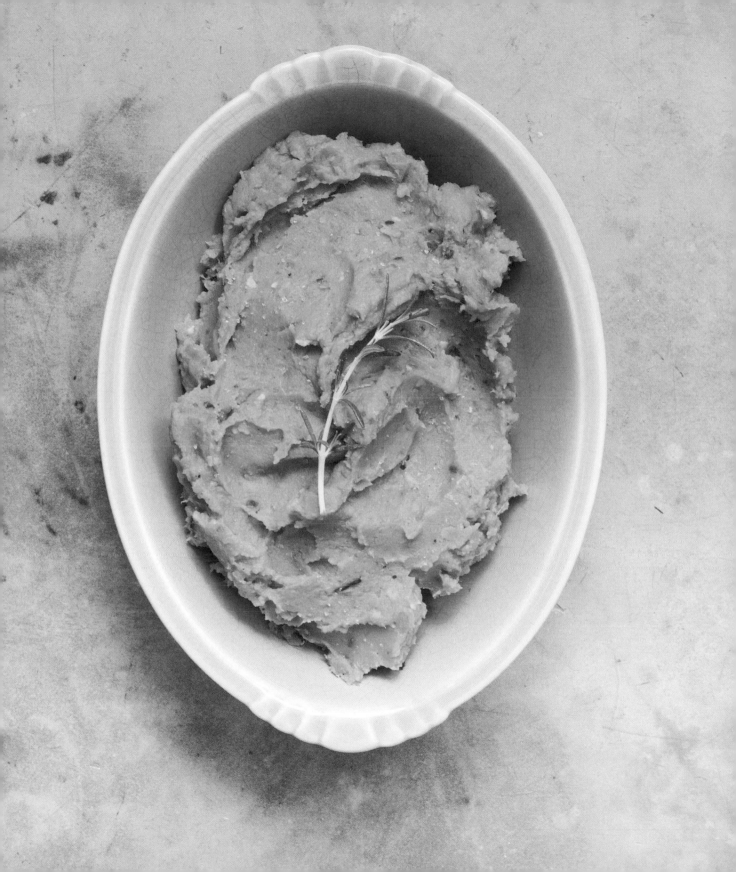

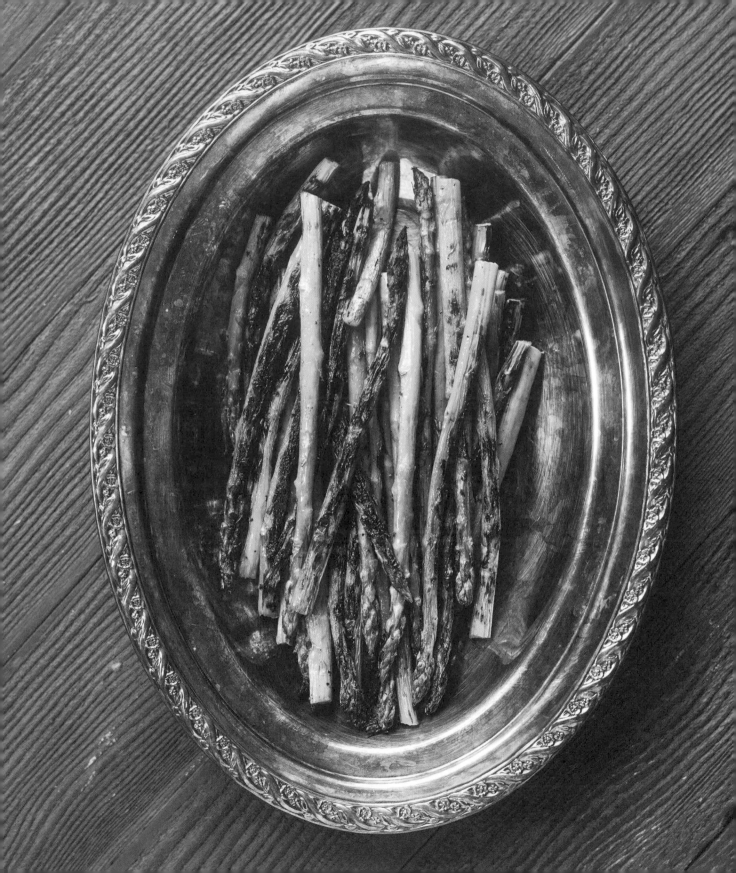

ROSEMARY GRILLED ASPARAGUS

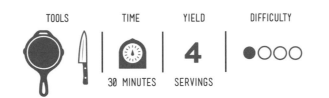

TOOLS   TIME   YIELD   DIFFICULTY

30 MINUTES   4 SERVINGS   ●○○○

900 g asparagus, rinsed and dried, ends trimmed

2 tablespoons solid cooking fat, melted

½ tablespoon minced fresh rosemary

¼ teaspoon sea salt

½ lemon, for finishing

1 Preheat your barbecue or griddle pan.

2 Coat the asparagus evenly with the cooking fat, rosemary and salt.

3 Grill for 10 minutes or until soft, turning occasionally, removing some of the thinner spears as they cook. Serve warm with a squeeze of fresh lemon juice.

Variation: You can also roast these for 10 to 12 minutes in a 200°C oven.

Storage: Keeps well in the refrigerator for several days (although the asparagus may turn a duller shade of green due to the acidic properties of the lemon juice).

Serving Suggestions: Rainbow Roasted Root Vegetables (page 188), Lemon-Garlic Marinated Grilled Chicken (page 219), Herbed Roast Chicken (page 227), Citrus-Ginger Salmon (page 237), Herbed Dry-Rub Steak (page 265)

PURÉED PARSNIPS

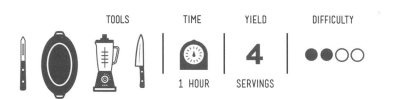

TOOLS TIME YIELD DIFFICULTY

4
1 HOUR SERVICES ●●○○

900 g parsnips, peeled and
  chopped into chunks
2 tablespoons solid cooking fat,
  melted, plus more as needed
¼ teaspoon sea salt

1 Preheat the oven to 200°C.

2 Place the parsnips in a bowl and toss to coat evenly with the cooking
fat and salt.

3 Place in a baking dish and cook in the oven for 1 hour or until soft, stirring
a couple of times while cooking.

4 Purée in a high-powered blender or food processor until the desired
consistency is reached (you may like the puréed parsnips a bit on the chunky
side or very smooth), adding more fat if necessary. Serve warm.

Storage: Keeps in the refrigerator for several days.

Serving Suggestions: Brussels Sprouts with Crispy Bacon (page 191), Sage-Braised
Chicken Legs (page 228), Cranberry-Braised Beef Short Ribs (page 258),
Braised Lamb Shanks (page 273), Lamb Chops (page 281)

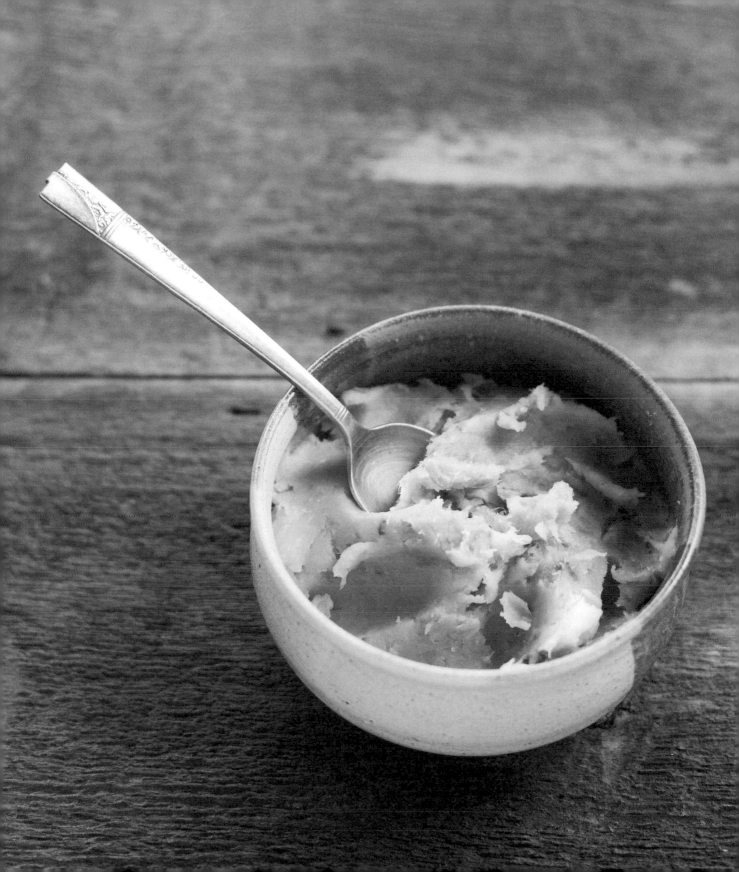

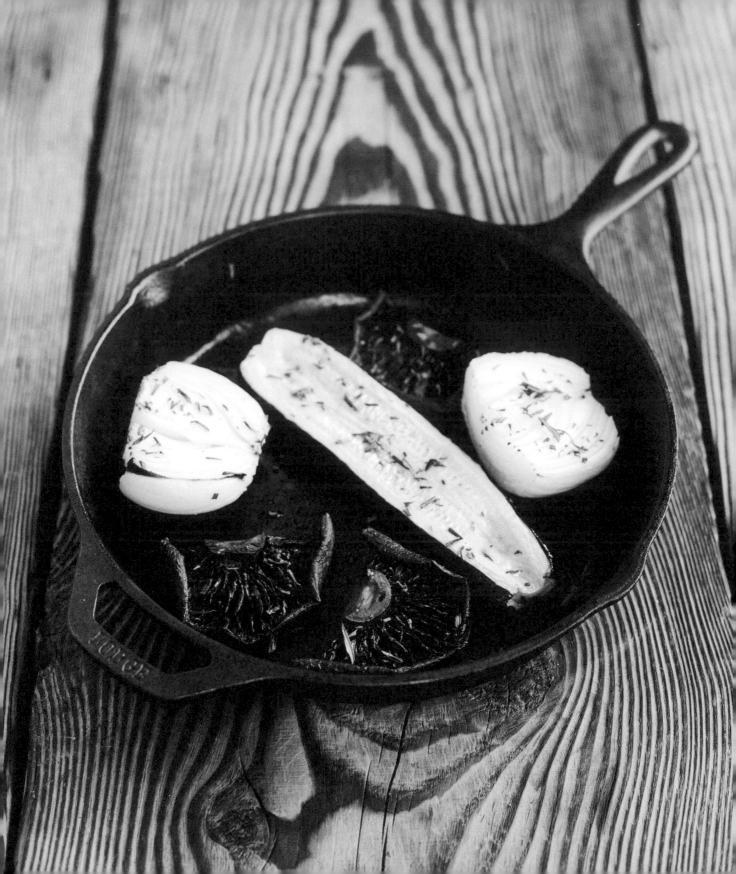

ROASTED MIXED VEGETABLES

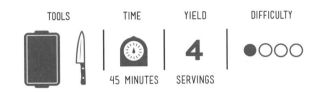

TOOLS | TIME | YIELD | DIFFICULTY

45 MINUTES | 4 SERVINGS | ●○○○

1 large onion, peeled and quartered

4 courgettes (zucchini), cut in half lengthwise

2 portobello mushrooms, stalks removed and caps halved

2 tablespoons solid cooking fat, melted

1 tablespoon minced fresh rosemary

Sea salt to taste

1 Preheat the oven to 200°C.

2 Place the onion, courgette halves and mushrooms in a bowl and coat evenly with the cooking fat, rosemary and salt.

3 Spread on a baking tray and cook in the oven for 30 minutes or until vegetables are tender and the outsides are caramelised. Serve warm.

Storage: Keeps in the refrigerator for several days.

Serving Suggestions: Chicken and Pesto Sauté (page 216), Herbed Roast Chicken (page 227), Mediterranean Salmon (page 242), Sole Fillet with Tarragon-Caper Sauce (page 245), Herb Stuffed Trout (page 253), Cranberry-Braised Beef Short Ribs (page 258), Braised Lamb Shanks (page 273), 'Spaghetti' and Meatballs (page 282)

CAULIFLOWER 'FRIED RICE'

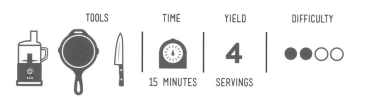

TOOLS   TIME   YIELD   DIFFICULTY

15 MINUTES   **4** SERVINGS   ●●○○

1 small head cauliflower, stem removed and head roughly chopped

2 tablespoons solid cooking fat

1 small onion, finely chopped

4 cloves garlic, minced

1 carrot, finely chopped

1 courgette (zucchini), finely chopped

90 g mushrooms, finely chopped

¼ teaspoon sea salt

½ teaspoon ground ginger

½ teaspoon ground turmeric

1 tablespoon coconut aminos

1 tablespoon chopped chives, for garnish

1 Process the cauliflower in a food processor for 10 seconds, or until it just barely forms rice-size granules; set aside.

2 Heat the cooking fat in the bottom of a large frying pan or wok on medium–high heat. When the fat has melted and the pan is hot, add the onion and cook for 5 minutes, stirring. Add the garlic and cook for a couple of minutes, until fragrant. Add the carrot and courgette and cook for another 5 minutes, stirring.

3 Add the cauliflower 'rice', mushrooms, salt, ginger, turmeric and coconut aminos, and cook 5 to 10 more minutes, stirring, until the vegetables are all soft. Serve garnished with chives.

Storage: Keeps in the refrigerator for several days.

Serving Suggestions: Asian-Marinated Grilled Chicken (page 219), Chicken Stir-Fry (page 231), Citrus-Ginger Marinated Salmon (page 237), Sear-Roasted Halibut (page 246), Shrimp and Green Bean Stir-Fry (page 249), Garlic Beef and Broccoli (page 270)

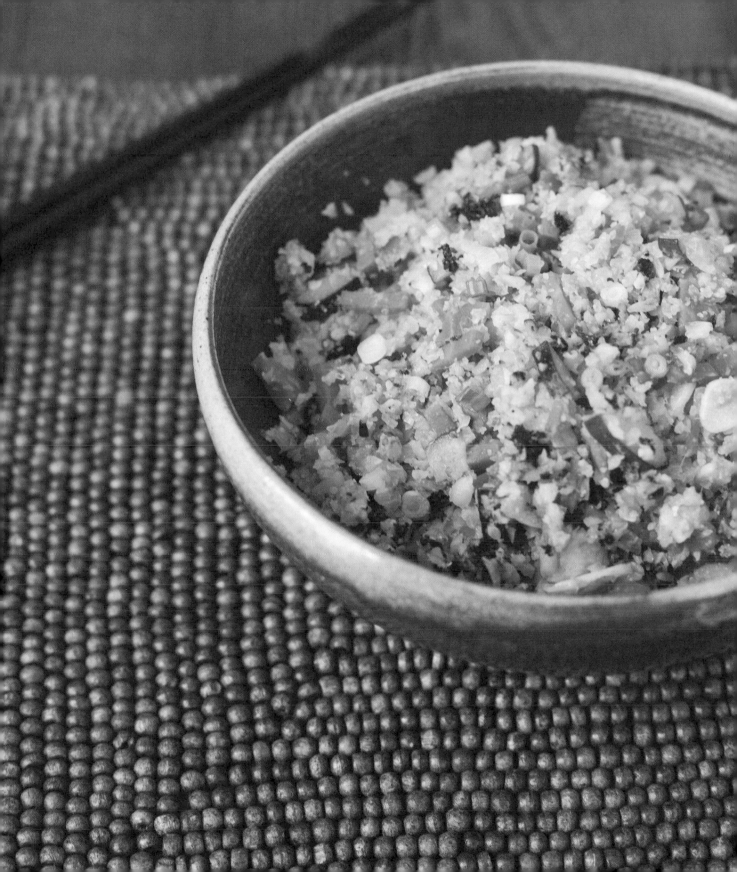

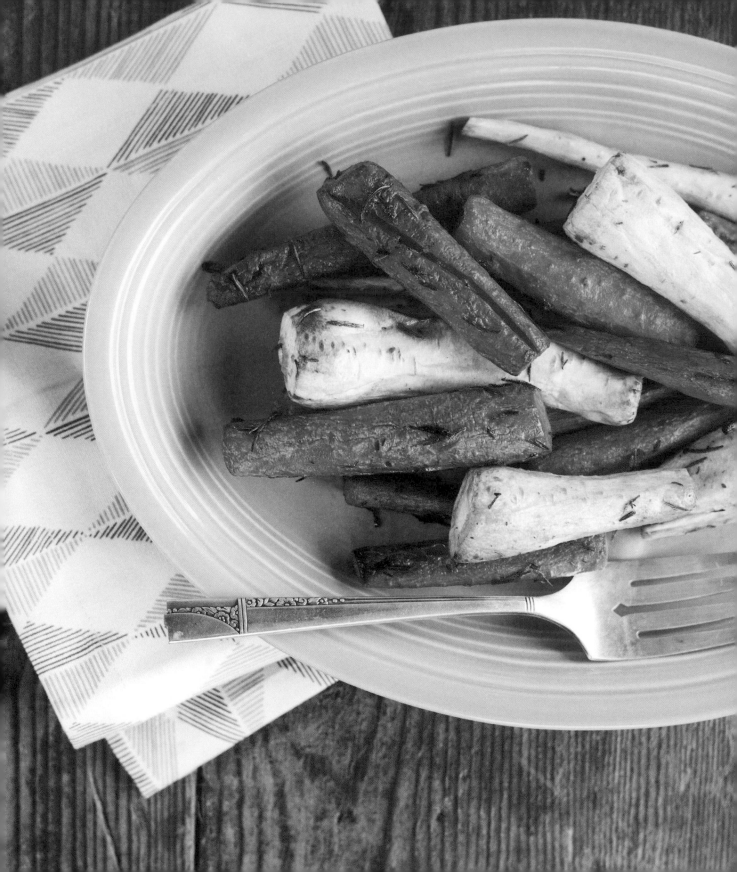

ROSEMARY-ROASTED CARROTS AND PARSNIPS

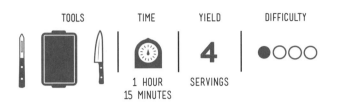

TOOLS	TIME	YIELD	DIFFICULTY
	1 HOUR 15 MINUTES	**4** SERVINGS	●○○○

450 g carrots, peeled and ends trimmed

225 g parsnips, peeled and ends trimmed

2 tablespoons solid cooking fat, melted

2 tablespoons minced fresh rosemary

Sea salt, to taste

1 Preheat the oven to 200°C.

2 Place the carrots and parsnips in a large baking dish then add the cooking fat, rosemary and salt and toss lightly to coat the vegetables evenly.

3 Cook for about 1 hour, stirring every 20 minutes to ensure even browning. The vegetables are finished when tender and lightly caramelised on the outside.

Storage: Keeps in the refrigerator for several days.

Serving Suggestions: Sautéed Market Greens (page 183), Garlic-Sage Chicken Patties (page 211), Herbed Roast Chicken (page 227), Sage-Braised Chicken Legs (page 228), Stuffed Whole Trout (page 253), Cranberry-Braised Beef Short Ribs (page 258), Citrus-Thyme Pot Roast (page 266)

SEARED BROCCOLINI
WITH COCONUT-BASIL PESTO

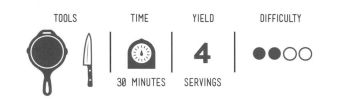

TOOLS	TIME	YIELD	DIFFICULTY
	30 MINUTES	4 SERVINGS	●●○○

2 tablespoons solid cooking fat

450 g broccolini, washed, ends of stems removed

4 cloves garlic, minced

250 ml Coconut-Basil Pesto (page 124)

1 Heat the cooking fat in a large frying pan on high heat. When the fat has melted and the pan is hot, sear the broccolini for a couple of minutes on each side. Turn the heat down to medium, add the garlic and let cook, covered, for about 10 minutes, or until the broccolini is tender.

2 Serve with coconut pesto drizzled over the top.

Storage: Keeps well in the refrigerator.

Serving Suggestions: Curried Cauliflower (page 187), Puréed Parsnips (page 196), Herbed Roast Chicken (page 227)

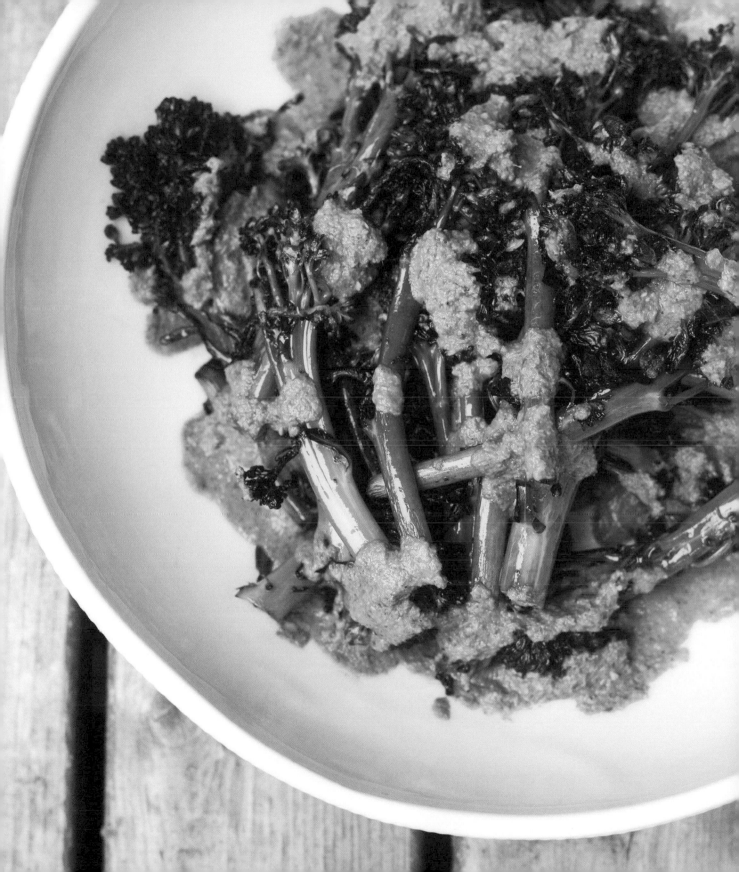

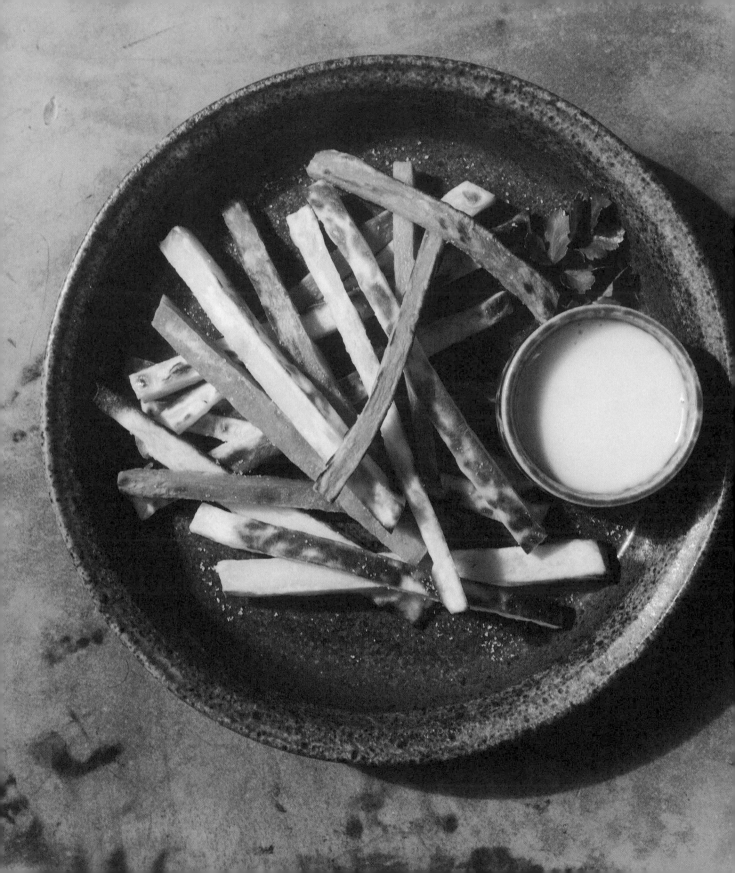

SWEET POTATO CHIPS WITH GARLIC 'MAYO'

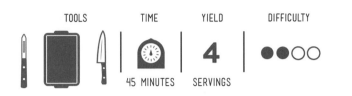

TOOLS	TIME	YIELD	DIFFICULTY
	45 MINUTES	4 SERVINGS	●●○○

3 large sweet potatoes, peeled and cut into 1 cm-thick chips
60 ml solid cooking fat, melted
Sea salt
125 ml Garlic 'Mayo' (page 127)

1 Preheat the oven to 200°C.

2 Place the sweet potato chips in a large bowl and coat with the cooking fat and salt. Arrange on a few baking trays, making sure that the chips have adequate space between them (this is what makes them crispy!). Use 3 or 4 baking trays if you need to.

3 Bake for 10 minutes, remove from the oven, flip, and bake for another 10 to 15 minutes, watching at the end so that they don't burn.

4 Sprinkle with sea salt to taste and serve with the garlic 'mayo'.

Serving Suggestions: Garlic-Sage Chicken Patties (page 211), Three-Herb Beef Patties (page 262), Portobello 'Burger' (page 274), Cinnamon-Sage Dry Rubbed Steak (page 265)

POULTRY

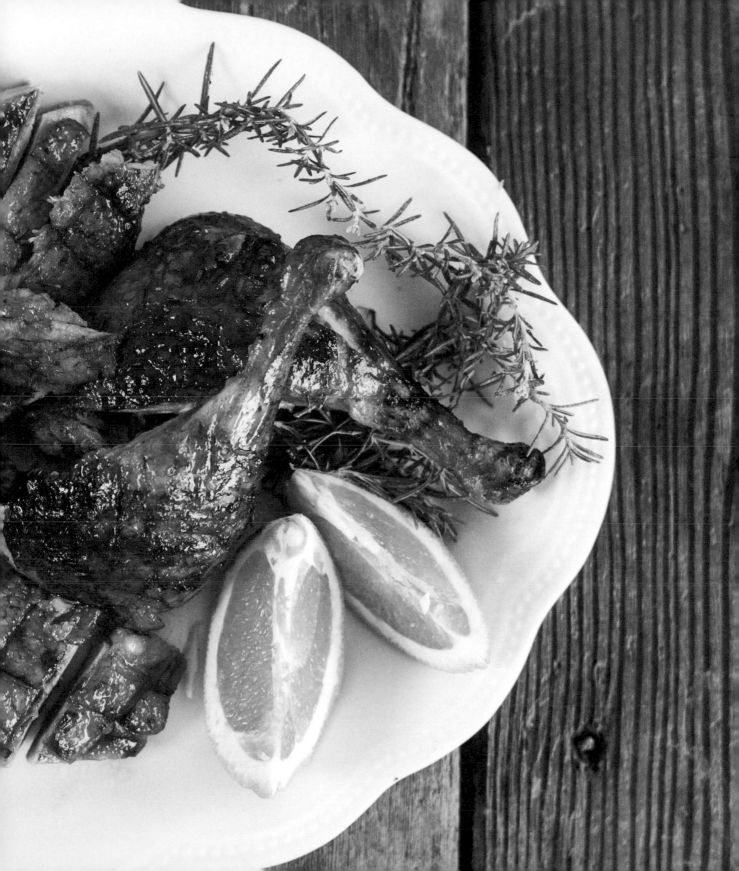

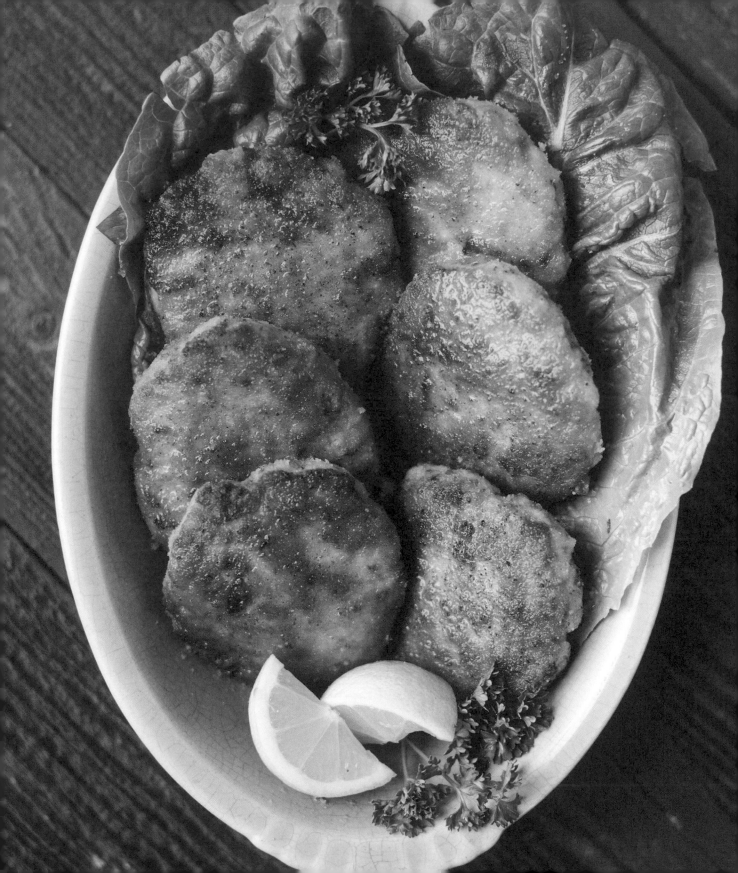

GARLIC-SAGE
CHICKEN PATTIES

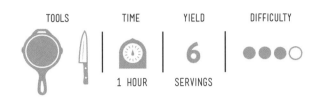

TOOLS   TIME   YIELD   DIFFICULTY

6

1 HOUR   SERVINGS

●●●○

4 tablespoons solid cooking fat

40 g minced onion

4 cloves garlic, minced

3 tablespoons chopped fresh sage

4 tablespoons coconut flour,
    plus 1 tablespoon, divided

900 g free-range chicken thighs,
    minced

1 teaspoon sea salt

1 Heat 1 tablespoon of the cooking fat in a frying pan on medium heat. When the fat has melted and the pan is hot, add the onion and cook for about 5 minutes, stirring, until soft. Add the garlic and sage and continue to cook for a couple of minutes, until the mixture is fragrant.

2 Take the pan off the heat and let the mixture cool. While you are waiting, place the 30 g of coconut flour on a plate.

3 When the onion mixture is no longer hot, add it to the minced chicken, along with the 1 tablespoon coconut flour and the salt. Mix well, then form into 12 to 14 patties. Dredge them lightly in the coconut flour on the plate.

4 Reheat the frying pan over medium heat, adding more cooking fat if there isn't any left in the pan. Cook the patties in batches for 10 to 15 minutes per side, until golden brown and completely cooked throughout.

Variation: If you don't want to cook the chicken patties on the stovetop, they can be baked in the oven for about 25 minutes at 200°C. You can also try forming them into meatballs instead of patties. Brown in a frying pan with some coconut oil until the meatballs firm up, then add 125 ml of bone broth, cover, and simmer until completely cooked (another 10 minutes or so).

Storage: Keeps in the refrigerator for several days. Also freezes well.

Serving Suggestions: Sautéed Market Greens (page 183), Mashed Sweet Potatoes (page 192), Rosemary Grilled Asparagus (page 195)

SHREDDED CHICKEN BREAST

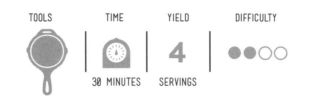

TOOLS TIME YIELD DIFFICULTY

30 MINUTES 4 SERVINGS

900 g free-range chicken breasts, skin on

¼ teaspoon sea salt

2 tablespoons solid cooking fat

250 ml Bone Broth (page 34) or water

1 Rinse the chicken breasts with cold water and pat dry. Bring to room temperature and sprinkle them with the salt.

2 Heat the cooking fat in a frying pan over medium heat.

3 When the fat is melted and the pan is hot, place the chicken, skin-side down, and cook for 5 to 7 minutes, or until browned. Flip the chicken, add the broth, cover, and lower the heat to a simmer. Cook for about 20 minutes, or until the internal temperature reaches 75°C.

4 Let cool, discard the skin then shred the meat for use in all sorts of wonderful dishes!

Storage: Keeps for several days in the refrigerator.

Serving Suggestions: Serve in lettuce cups (whole lettuce leaves) or as a salad with Mango Salsa (page 131) and Guacamole (page 128).

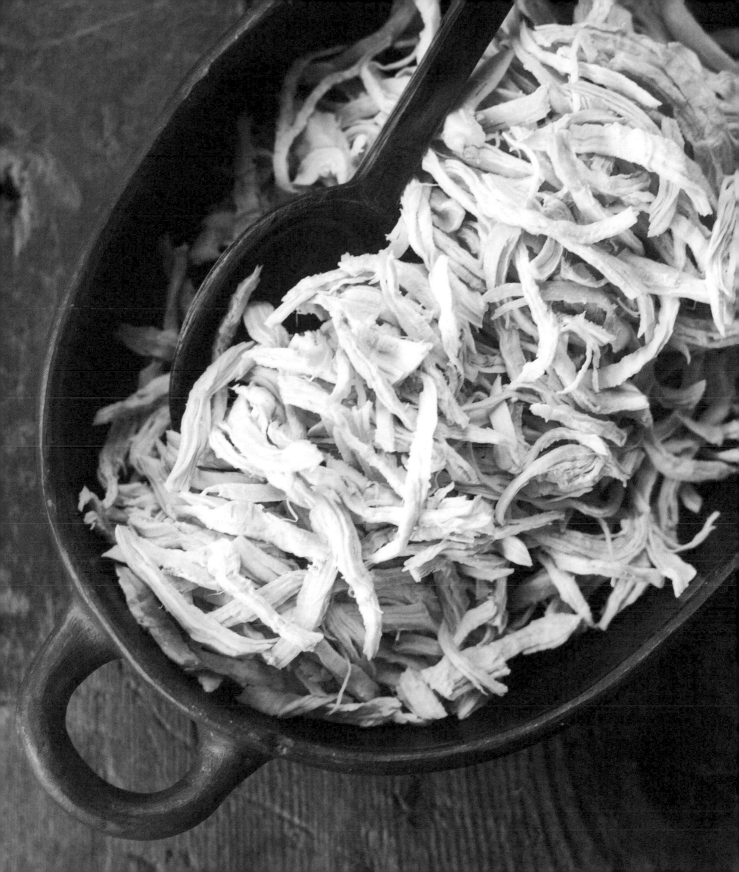

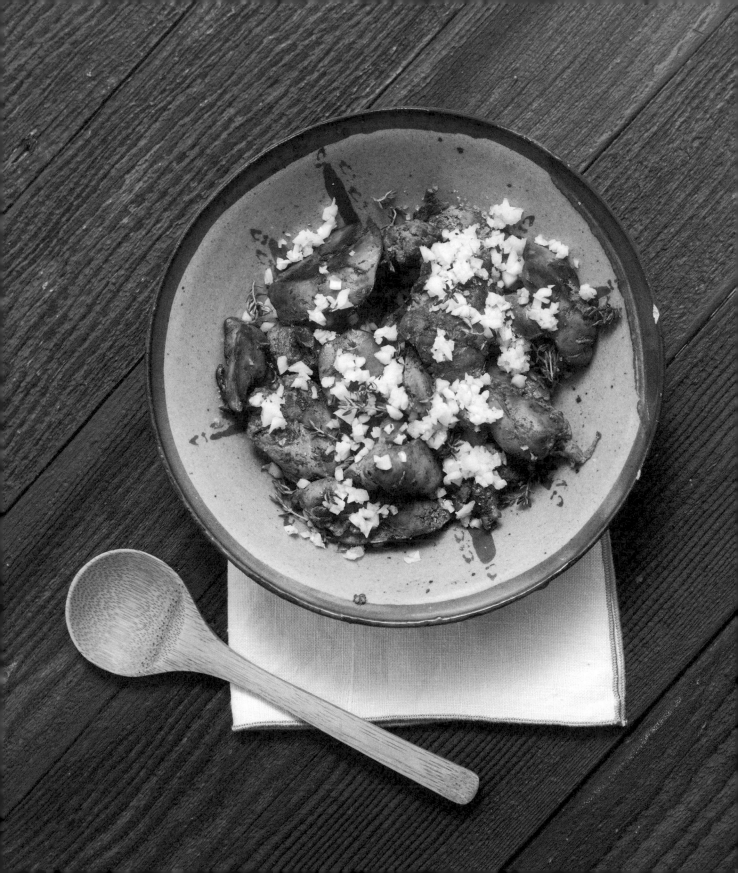

CHICKEN LIVER WITH RAW GARLIC AND THYME

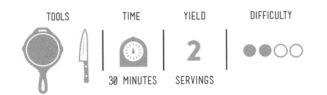

TOOLS TIME YIELD DIFFICULTY

30 MINUTES 2 SERVINGS ●●○○

450 g free-range chicken livers
3 tablespoons extra-virgin
 olive oil
1 lemon, juiced
 (about 2 tablespoons)
4 cloves garlic, minced
¼ teaspoon sea salt
Fresh thyme, for garnish

1 Prepare the livers by washing and drying them thoroughly. You want them to be as dry as possible before cooking to make sure they get nice and crispy.

2 Heat a frying pan on medium-high, and when it is hot, dry-fry the livers for 3 to 4 minutes before flipping. Cook for another 2 to 3 minutes on the other side. They are done cooking when they are fully brown and no longer pink inside (you can cut one open to check).

3 Remove from the pan and coat with olive oil, lemon juice, raw garlic, salt and thyme. Serve warm.

Storage: Keeps in the refrigerator for several days.

Serving Suggestions: Sautéed Market Greens (page 183), Rainbow Roasted Root Vegetables (page 188)

CHICKEN AND PESTO SAUTÉ

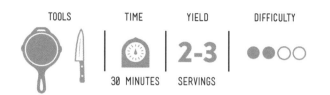

TOOLS | TIME | YIELD | DIFFICULTY

30 MINUTES | 2-3 SERVINGS | ●●○○

2 tablespoons solid cooking fat

450 g broccolini, roughly chopped

450 g shredded chicken breast meat (page 212)

250 ml Coconut-Basil Pesto (page 124)

1 Heat the cooking fat in the bottom of a large cast-iron pan or frying pan on medium heat. When the fat has melted and the pan is hot, add the broccolini, cover, and cook for 10 to 15 minutes, stirring occasionally.

2 Add the shredded chicken and coconut pesto and stir to combine. Cook for another minute or two until everything is incorporated.

Variation: Feel free to use broccoli if broccolini is not available to you.

Storage: Keeps in the refrigerator for several days.

Serving Suggestions: Serve on a bed of courgette (zucchini) noodles, cooked spaghetti squash or with Roast Mixed Vegetables (page 199).

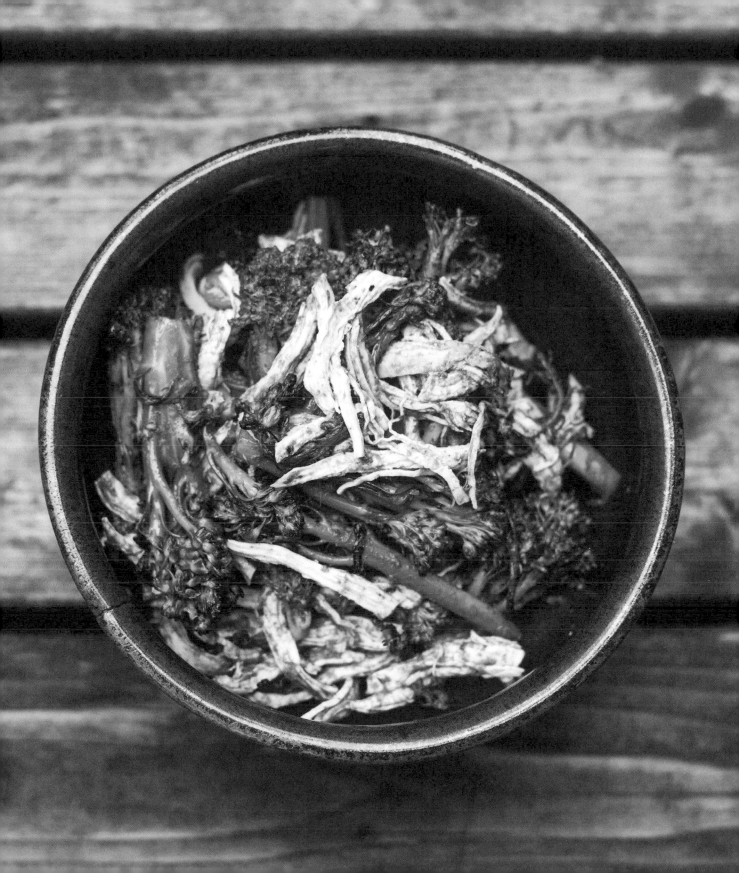

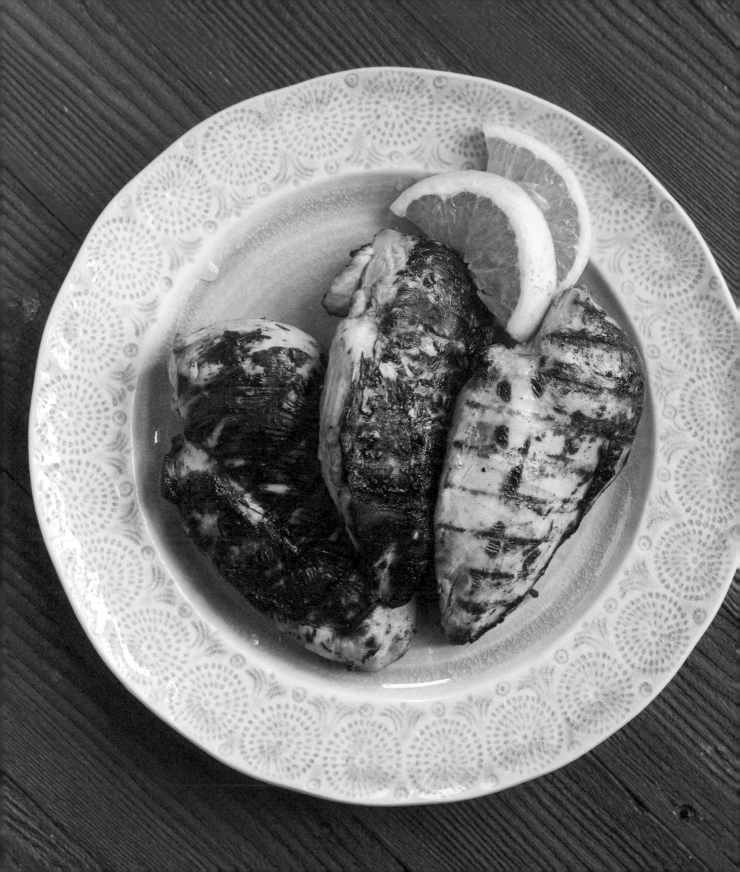

MARINATED
GRILLED CHICKEN

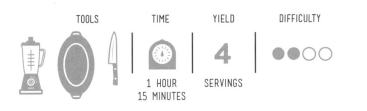

TOOLS	TIME	YIELD	DIFFICULTY
	1 HOUR 15 MINUTES	4 SERVINGS	●●○○

680 g free-range chicken
  breasts, butterflied
1 tablespoon solid cooking fat

Asian Marinade Variation:
60 ml coconut aminos
1 orange, juiced (about 80 ml)
2.5 cm piece ginger, peeled
  and minced
1 clove garlic, minced
¼ teaspoon sea salt

Lemon-Garlic
Marinade Variation:
2 lemons, juiced (about 60 ml)
2 cloves garlic, minced
2 tablespoons minced
  fresh parsley
½ teaspoon sea salt

1 Choose which variation of the marinade you are going to make. Combine the ingredients in a blender and blend for 30 seconds.

2 Pour the marinade into a bag or container with the chicken and marinate for 1 to 2 hours, turning halfway through if the chicken is not completely covered in the marinade.

3 When it is time to cook the chicken, brush your barbecue or griddle pan with the cooking fat and heat to a medium–high heat.

4 Remove the chicken, pat dry, and discard the remaining marinade. Cook for about 10 minutes per side, or until the chicken is cooked throughout. Alternatively, bake the chicken in the oven at 200°C for about 30 minutes.

Storage: Keeps in the refrigerator for several days.

Serving Suggestions: Rosemary Grilled Asparagus (page 195), Cauliflower 'Fried Rice' (page 200)

ORANGE-ROSEMARY DUCK

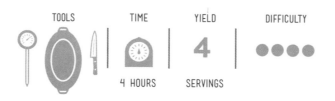

TOOLS | TIME | YIELD | DIFFICULTY

4 HOURS

4 SERVINGS

●●●●

1 x 2.25 kg free-range duck

5 oranges, juiced and strained (about 250 ml)

2 tablespoons maple syrup

1 tablespoon minced fresh rosemary

1 teaspoon sea salt

1 Preheat the oven to 140°C.

2 Rinse the duck with cool water and dry it thoroughly. Cut off the excess skin around the cavity and neck, saving it to render later if desired. Cut a cross-hatch pattern through the skin (being careful not to slice the meat underneath) anywhere there is a lot of fat—particularly around the breast, sides and thighs of the bird. Make sure the slices are about 2.5 cm apart from each other. Fold the wings under and, using kitchen twine, truss the legs together. Place the duck breast-side up on a rack set in a shallow roasting tin.

3 Cook the duck for 45 minutes, removing it once halfway through cooking to prick it all over with a sharp knife. The goal of the pricking is to make little holes for the fat to drain out of, so do this wherever there is a lot of fat.

4 Turn the duck so that it is breast-side down and cook for another 45 minutes, removing it once more halfway through to prick the fat. If there is a lot of liquid fat in the bottom of the tin, transfer the duck to another tin while you pour the fat into a jar for future use.

5 Remove the duck, prick the fat and cook for another 45 minutes, breast-side up, removing another time halfway through to prick the fat.

6 Remove the duck, prick the fat and cook for another 45 minutes breast down, removing another time halfway through to prick the fat. At this point, the bird will have been in the oven for 3 hours. Measure the internal temperature, and if it is not at 75°C measured at the inside of the thigh, continue cooking until it reaches that temperature.

7 While the duck is in the oven for the last time, bring the orange juice, maple syrup, rosemary and salt to a boil in a small saucepan. Reduce the heat to a simmer, and cook for about 20 minutes, until the mixture has reduced to a thick glaze.

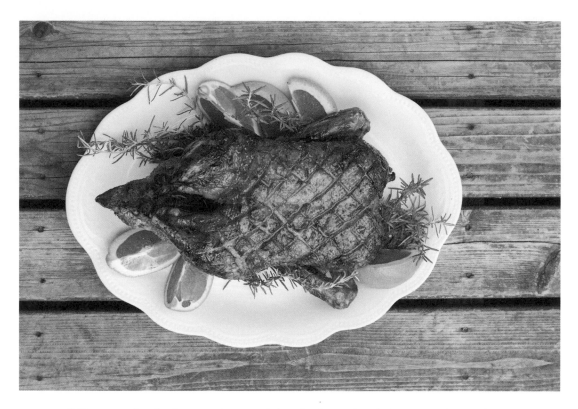

8 Remove the duck, pour the remaining fat from the tin into your jar, and turn the oven up to 200°C. Prick the fat one last time. Using a pastry brush, glaze the entire bird with the orange-rosemary mixture. Cook for a final 5 to 10 minutes, breast up, until the glaze turns a deep mahogany brown (watch closely to make sure it doesn't burn).

9 Let the duck rest, loosely covered, for 20 minutes. Carve and serve.

Note: It is best to clean and dry the duck at least a few hours before cooking, if not the day before—store it in the refrigerator, uncovered, to give it plenty of time to dry. This will help ensure the skin comes out nice and crispy. Duck fat is one of the most flavourful fats to cook with, and tastes wonderful with roasted root vegetables. To render the extra fat, cut the pieces of fat and skin into small pieces and place them in a small saucepan with a couple tablespoons of water. Simmer until all of the water has evaporated, most of the fat has rendered and the skin is crispy. Strain and pour the fat into a jar for future use.

Storage: Rendered duck fat can be stored in the fridge for a couple of months. Cooked duck keeps for several days in the refrigerator.

Serving Suggestions: Cabbage Slaw with Olive-Avocado Dressing (page 145), Citrus-Spinach Salad (page 150), Carrot-Ginger Soup (page 162), Rainbow Roasted Root Vegetables (page 188), Rosemary-Roasted Carrots and Parsnips (page 203)

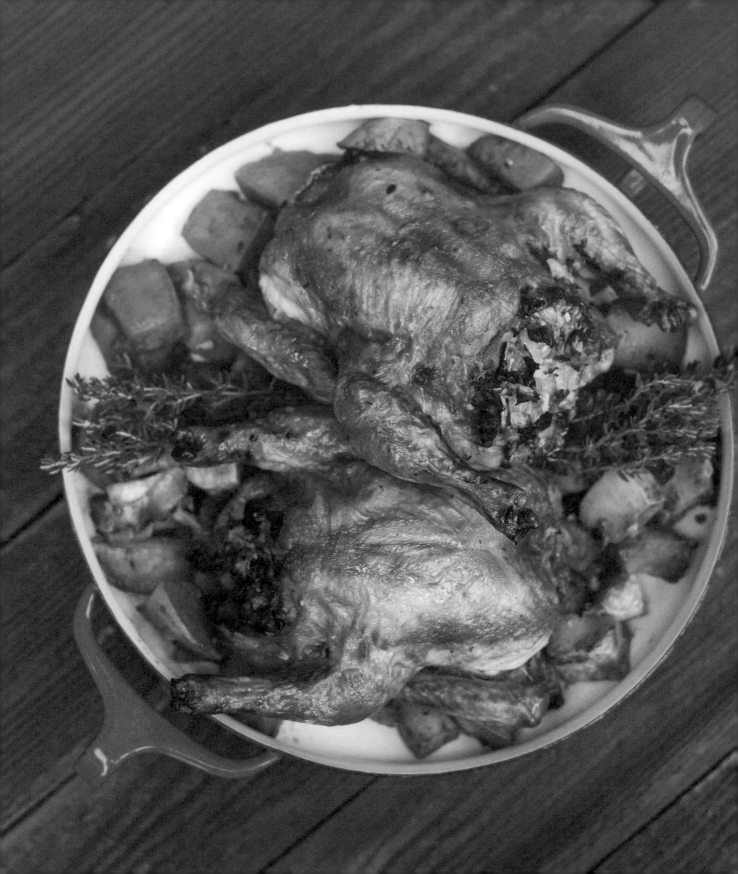

MUSHROOM-STUFFED CORNISH HENS

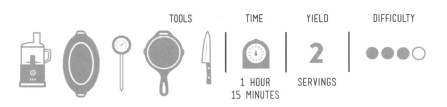

TOOLS   TIME   YIELD   DIFFICULTY

1 HOUR 15 MINUTES

2 SERVINGS

●●●○

1 tablespoon solid cooking fat

½ onion, finely chopped

2 cloves garlic, minced

125 g cauliflower, riced*

90 g finely chopped crimini mushrooms

1 tablespoons chopped fresh thyme

¼ teaspoon sea salt, plus more for seasoning

1 large sweet potato, cut into 4 cm chunks

2 free-range Cornish game hens

½ lemon, juiced (about 1 tablespoon)

1 Preheat the oven to 200°C.

2 Heat the cooking fat in a frying pan on medium heat. When the fat has melted and the pan is hot, add the onion and cook for 5 minutes, stirring. Add the garlic and cook another couple of minutes, stirring, until fragrant. Add the cauliflower, mushrooms, thyme, and the salt and cook, stirring for another 5 minutes, until softened but not completely cooked. Remove from heat and set aside to cool.

3 Lightly salt the sweet potatoes and place them in a small roasting tin.

4 Rinse the hens with cool water and thoroughly dry each one. Sprinkle sea salt inside the cavity and rub it all over the skin. Stuff the cavities with the cauliflower and mushroom mixture along with some lemon juice.

5 Arrange the game hens, breast-side up, on top of the sweet potatoes in the roasting tin. Roast for 1 hour, removing halfway through to rotate the hens so that the legs that were facing the outside are now facing in. Check to ensure they reach an internal temperature of 75°C when measured at the thickest portion of the inside of the thigh.

6 Serve one hen per person, on a bed of roasted sweet potatoes.

*Note: To make cauliflower 'rice', place the roughly chopped florets into a food processor and process lightly, until rice-size granules form.

Variation: Substitute another variety of starchy vegetable for the sweet potato, such as hard winter squash or parsnips.

Storage: Keeps in the refrigerator for several days.

Serving Suggestions: Market Salad (page 149), Citrus-Spinach Salad (page 150), Brussels Sprouts with Crispy Bacon (page 191), Sautéed Market Greens (page 183)

CURRIED CHICKEN SALAD

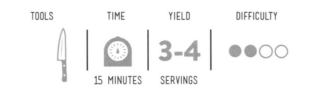

TOOLS	TIME	YIELD	DIFFICULTY
	15 MINUTES	**3-4** SERVINGS	●●○○

125 ml Garlic 'Mayo' (page 127)

1 teaspoon apple cider vinegar

½ lemon, juiced
(about 1 tablespoon)

2 teaspoons ground turmeric

1 teaspoon ground ginger

¼ teaspoon sea salt

450 g shredded chicken breast
meat (page 212)

40 g chopped red onion

45 g raisins

2 tablespoons chopped flat-leaf
parsley, for garnish

1 Soften the mayo in a warm water bath until it is a liquid.

2 Combine the mayo, vinegar, lemon juice, turmeric, ginger and salt in a large bowl and whisk to combine.

3 Add the chicken breast, red onion and raisins. Stir to combine. Serve garnished with chopped parsley.

Storage: Keeps in the refrigerator for several days.

Serving Suggestions: Market Salad (page 149), Citrus-Spinach Salad (page 150), Radish and Jicama Tabbouli (page 142)

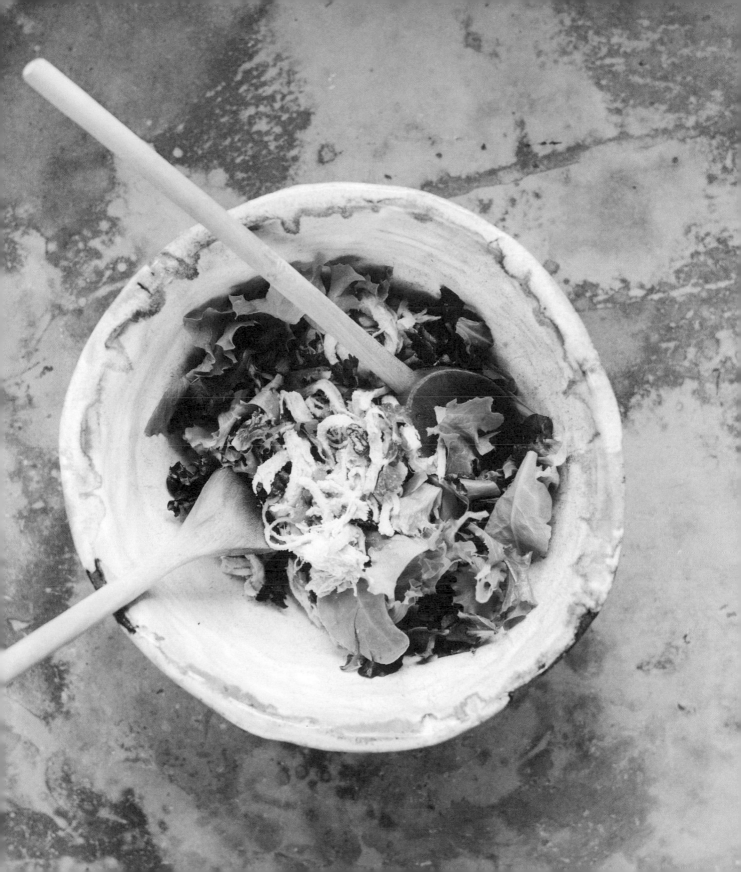

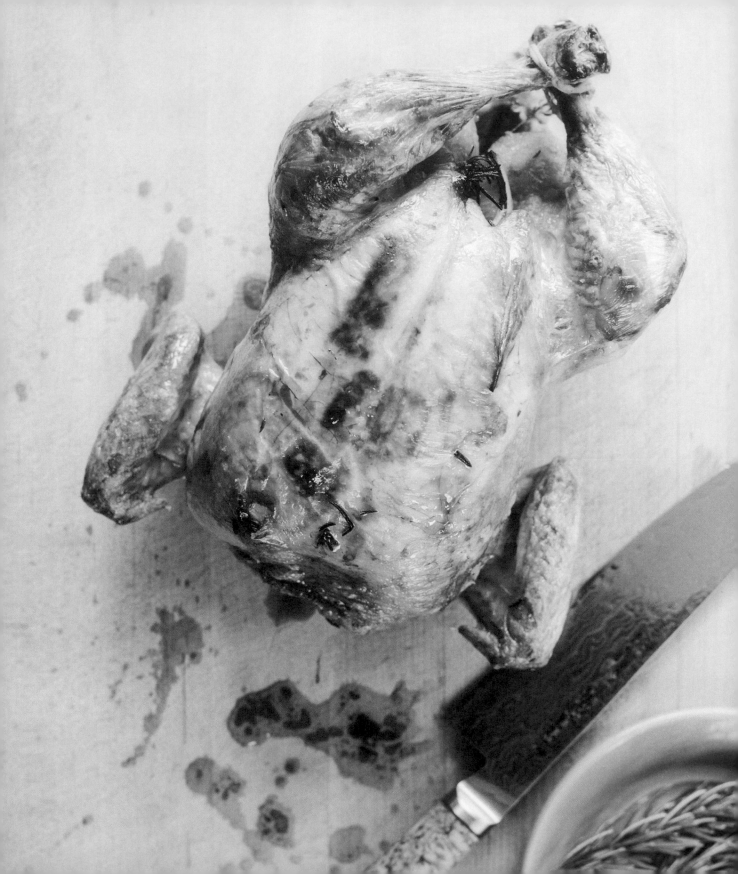

HERBED ROAST CHICKEN

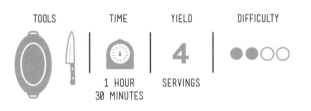

TOOLS	TIME	YIELD	DIFFICULTY
	1 HOUR 30 MINUTES	4 SERVINGS	●●○○

1 x 1.3–1.8 kg free-range chicken

Sea salt

A few sprigs of assorted fresh herbs (thyme, rosemary and sage work well)

4 cloves garlic, peeled and halved

1 lemon, quartered

1 Preheat the oven to 200°C.

2 Rinse the chicken with cool water and dry it thoroughly. Rub salt all over the inside and outside of the chicken. Place it breast-side up on a rack in a roasting tin. Place the sprigs of herbs and the garlic halves under the skin at the neck and the rear of the bird. Fill the cavity with the lemon quarters and any leftover herbs.

3 Cook for 20 minutes, breast-side up. Flip the chicken over, then cook for another 20 minutes, breast-side down. Flip once again and cook for a final 20 minutes, breast-side up. Check the internal temperature (measured at the thickest part of the thigh), and continue cooking if it is less than 75°C. Remove from the oven and let the chicken rest, lightly covered, for about 15 minutes before serving.

Note: If you don't have a rack, you can cook the chicken on top of a bed of carrots and celery.

Storage: Keeps in the refrigerator for several days.

Serving Suggestions: Brussels Sprouts with Crispy Bacon (page 191), Rainbow Roasted Root Vegetables (page 188), Puréed Parsnips (page 196), Roasted Mixed Vegetables (page 199), Sautéed Market Greens (page 183)

SAGE-BRAISED CHICKEN LEGS

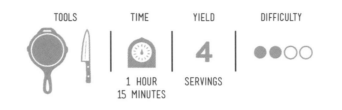

TOOLS	TIME	YIELD	DIFFICULTY
	1 HOUR 15 MINUTES	4 SERVINGS	●●○○

3–4 free-range whole chicken
    legs, skin on

2 tablespoons solid cooking fat

6 cloves garlic, chopped

180 g halved button or crimini
    mushrooms

A small handful chopped fresh
    sage

2 tablespoons apple cider vinegar

80 ml Bone Broth (page 34)

80 ml filtered water

¼ teaspoon sea salt

½ lemon, juiced
    (about 1 tablespoon)

1 Preheat the oven to 150°C.

2 Rinse the chicken legs with cool water and pat them dry. Make sure they are at room temperature before frying.

3 Heat the cooking fat in an ovenproof frying pan or cast-iron pan on medium–high heat. When the fat has melted and the pan is hot, brown the chicken, skin-side down, for 8 minutes, or until golden and crispy. Remove from the pan and set aside.

4 Turn the heat down to medium and add the garlic, stirring while cooking for a minute. Add the mushrooms and sage, cooking for another few minutes while stirring. Turn off the heat, add the apple cider vinegar and return the chicken to the pan, with the crispy browned skin facing up.

5 Add the bone broth, water and salt, and place the pan in the oven. Cook for 35 to 45 minutes, or until a thermometer placed in the thickest part of the thigh reads 75°C.

6 Serve with some of the pan juices and fresh lemon juice drizzled on top.

Storage: Keeps in the refrigerator for several days.

Serving Suggestions: Parsnip Purée (page 196), Mashed Sweet Potatoes (page 192)

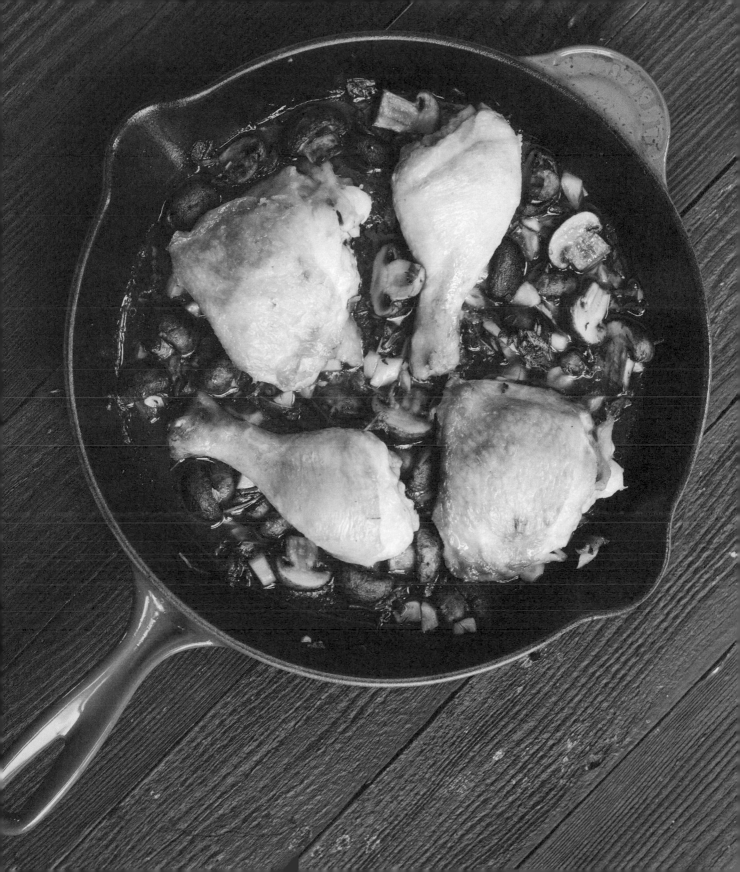

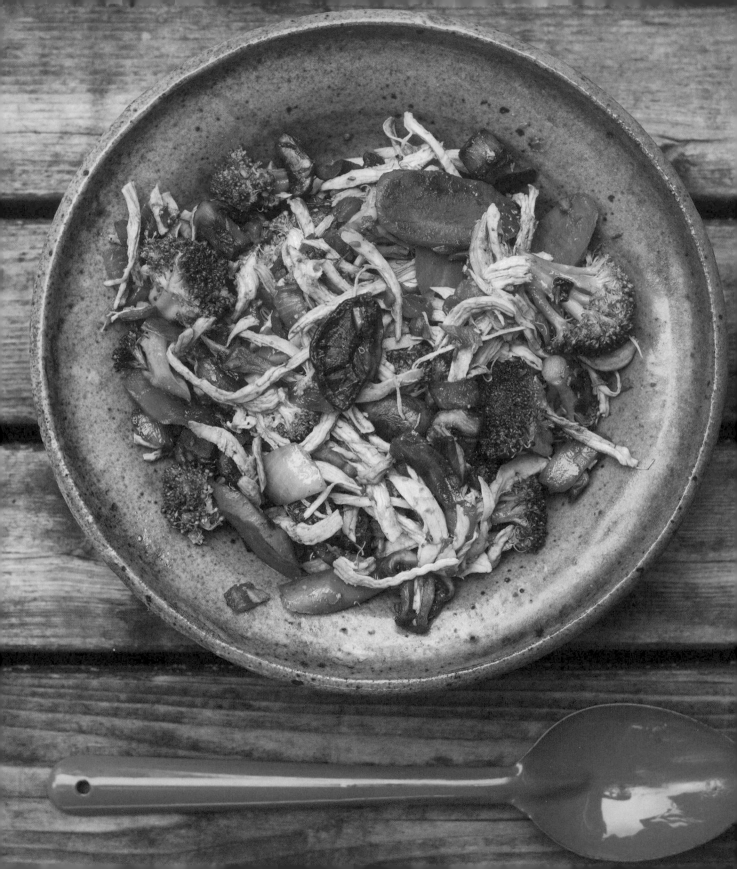

CHICKEN STIR-FRY

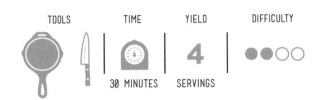

TOOLS | TIME | YIELD | DIFFICULTY

4

30 MINUTES | SERVINGS

● ● ○ ○

2 tablespoons solid cooking fat

1 onion, chopped

6 cloves garlic, minced

4 cm piece ginger, peeled
  and minced

3 large carrots, thinly sliced
  on the diagonal

450 g broccoli, chopped

½ teaspoon sea salt

125 ml coconut aminos

180 g chopped mushrooms

450 g shredded chicken breast
  meat (page 212)

½ lemon, juiced
  (about 1 tablespoon)

1 Heat the cooking fat in a wok or large frying pan on medium heat.

2 When the fat has melted and the pan is hot, add the onion and cook for 5 minutes, stirring. Add the garlic and ginger and cook, stirring for another minute. Add the carrot, broccoli, salt and coconut aminos and cover. Cook for 10 minutes, stirring occasionally. Add the mushrooms and cook for another 5 minutes. The vegetables should be firm yet cooked.

3 Add the chicken and stir to heat throughout. Drizzle over lemon juice and serve warm.

Storage: Keeps in the refrigerator for several days.

Serving Suggestions: Cauliflower 'Fried Rice' (page 200), Curried Cauliflower (page 187), Puréed Parsnips page 196)

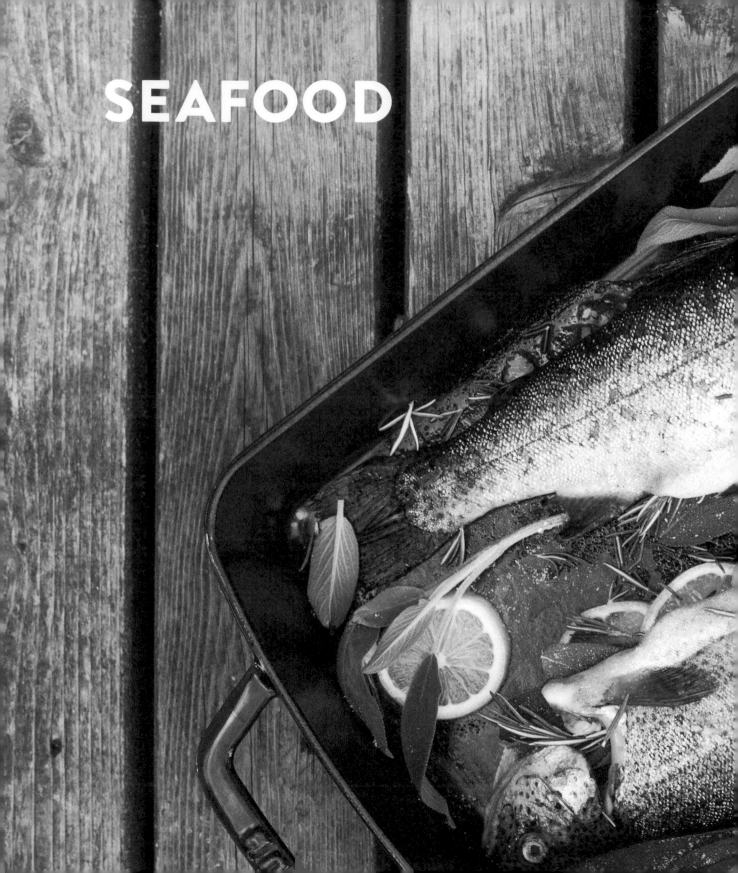

SEAFOOD

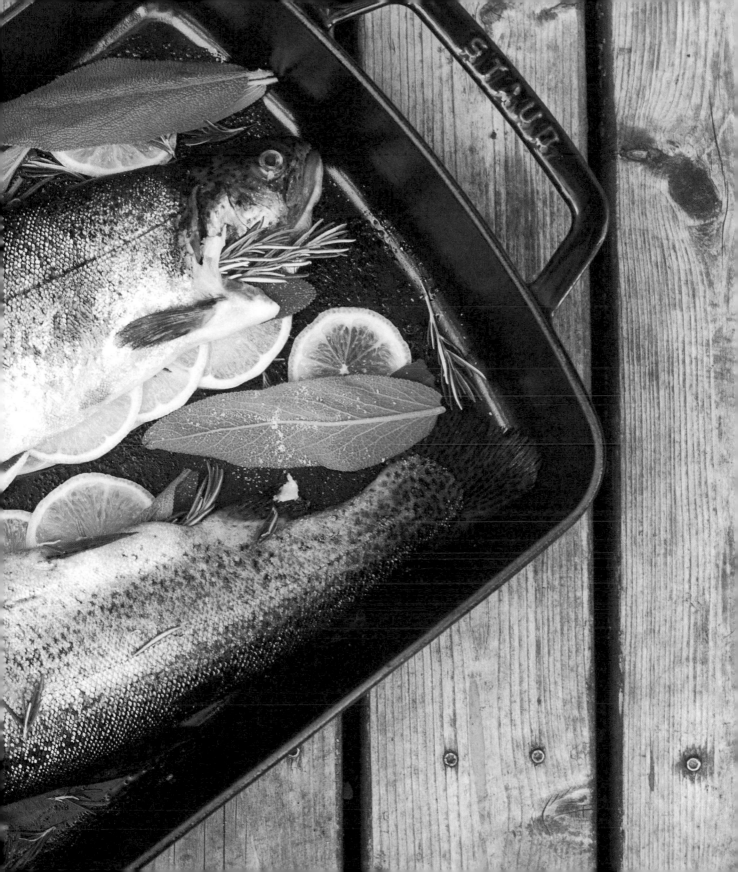

CLASSIC TUNA SALAD

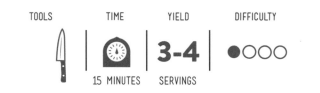

TOOLS	TIME	YIELD	DIFFICULTY
	15 MINUTES	3-4 SERVINGS	●○○○

185 ml Garlic 'Mayo' (page 127)
425 g BPA-free tinned tuna,
   drained
1 large carrot, finely chopped
1 celery stalk, finely chopped
3 tablespoons minced red onion
2 tablespoons minced fresh dill
½ lemon, juiced
   (about 1 tablespoon)
1 teaspoon apple cider vinegar
¼ teaspoon sea salt
Romaine lettuce, shredded or
   torn, for serving

1 Soften the mayo in a warm water bath until it is a liquid.

2 Combine the tuna, carrot, celery, red onion, dill, mayo, lemon juice, vinegar and salt in a bowl and mix to combine.

3 Serve on a bed of lettuce or in lettuce cups (whole lettuce leaves).

Storage: Keeps in the refrigerator for several days.

Serving Suggestions: Emerald Kale Salad (page 138), Citrus-Spinach Salad (page 150), Rainbow Roasted Root Vegetables (page 188)

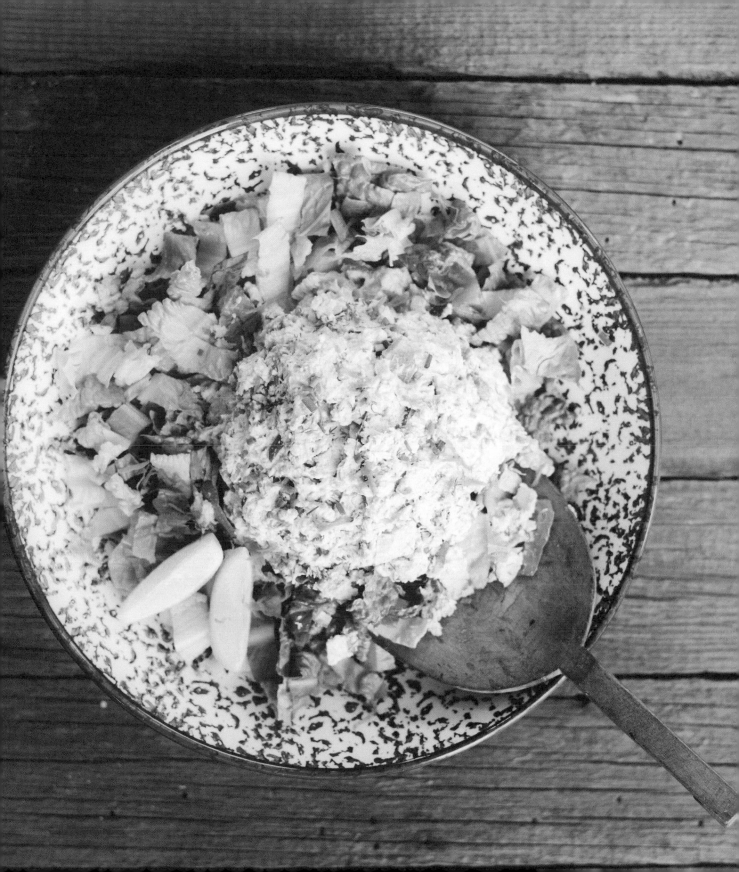

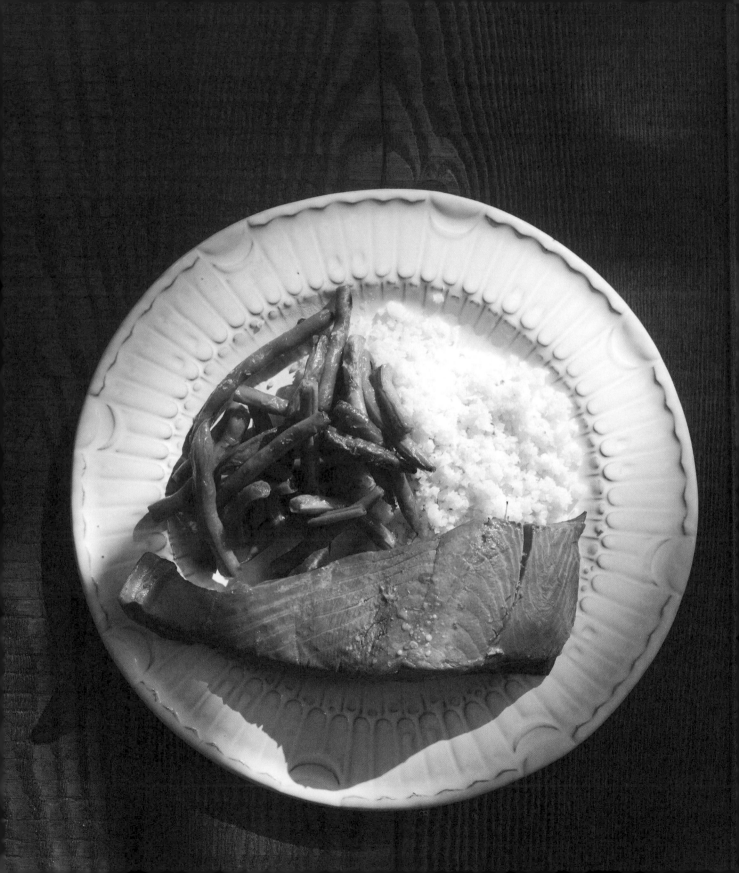

MARINATED SALMON

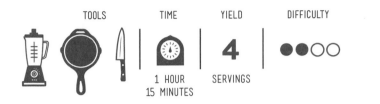

TOOLS   TIME   YIELD   DIFFICULTY

1 HOUR 15 MINUTES   4 SERVINGS

680 g wild-caught
   salmon fillets, skin on
   and deboned

Coconut Amino
Marinade Variation:
125 ml coconut aminos
1 lemon, juiced
   (about 2 tablespoons)
1 tablespoon chopped
   fresh thyme
¼ teaspoon ground ginger
¼ teaspoon sea salt

Citrus-Ginger
Marinade Variation:
2 oranges, juiced (about 170 ml)
1 tablespoon apple cider vinegar
1 tablespoon coconut aminos
   (optional)
2 tablespoons chopped
   fresh mint
2.5 cm piece ginger, peeled
¼ teaspoon sea salt

1 Place the salmon fillet in a large bag or container for marinating.

2 Choose which variation of marinade you will be making, and place all of the ingredients in a blender and blend for 30 seconds on high. Pour the marinade ingredients into the bag or container with the salmon and let marinate for 1 hour, flipping once or twice if the marinade doesn't completely cover the fish.

3 When you are ready to cook the salmon, preheat the oven to 200°C. Discard the marinade and place the salmon on an oiled baking tray, skin-side down. Bake for 15 minutes, or until the fish lightly flakes when tested with a fork. The cooking time may vary a bit depending on the thickness of your fish fillets.

Note: If you don't have a blender, just finely chop everything and whisk with the other marinade ingredients.

Storage: Keeps for a couple of days in the refrigerator.

Serving Suggestions: Cauliflower 'Fried Rice' (page 200), Curried Cauliflower (page 187), Market Salad (page 149)

SALMON SALAD WITH OLIVES AND CUCUMBER

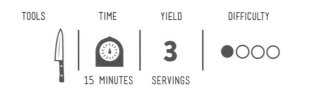

TOOLS | TIME | YIELD | DIFFICULTY

15 MINUTES | **3** SERVINGS | ●○○○

185 ml Garlic 'Mayo' (page 127)
½ lemon, juiced
   (about 1 tablespoon)
2 tablespoons olive oil
1 teaspoon apple cider vinegar
¼ teaspoon sea salt
425 g BPA-free tinned salmon,
   drained
½ cucumber, finely chopped
10 kalamata olives, pitted and
   finely chopped
4 radishes, minced (and an extra
   one finely sliced for garnish,
   if you like)
3 tablespoons minced red onion
2 tablespoons minced flat-leaf
   parsley
Mixed salad greens

1 Soften the mayo in a warm water bath until it is liquid.

2 Combine the mayo, lemon juice, olive oil, vinegar and salt in a large bowl.

3 Add the salmon, cucumber, olives, radishes, red onion and parsley and mix to combine.

4 Serve on a bed of mixed greens or in lettuce cups (whole lettuce leaves) with some slices of radish on top, if you like.

Storage: Keeps for a couple of days in the refrigerator.

Serving Suggestions: Olive Tapenade (page 91), Parsley-Garlic Dip (page 96), Emerald Kale Salad (page 138), Radish and Jicama Tabbouli (page 142)

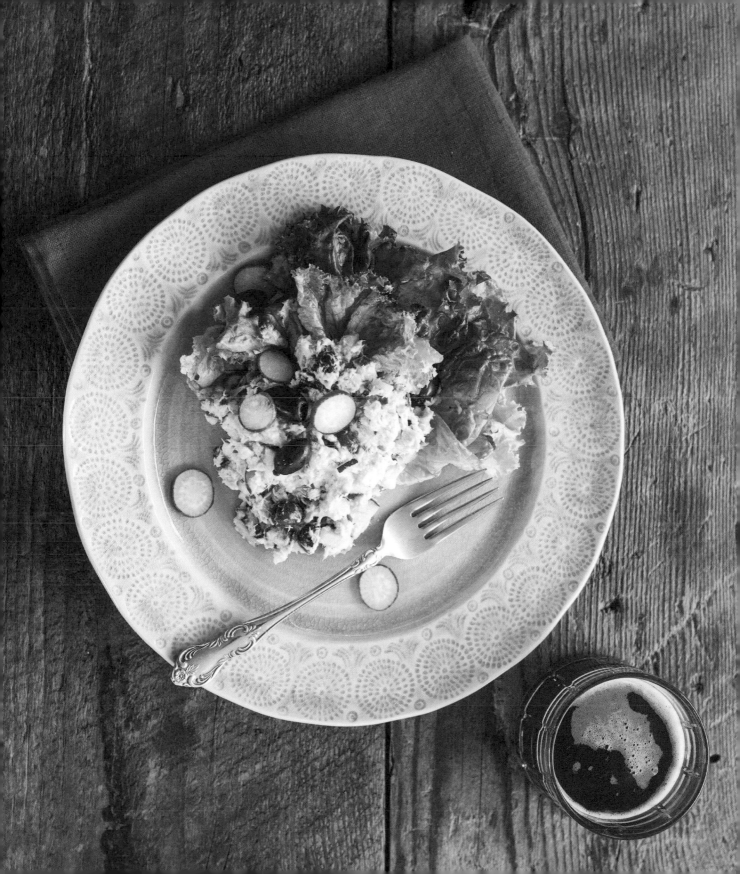

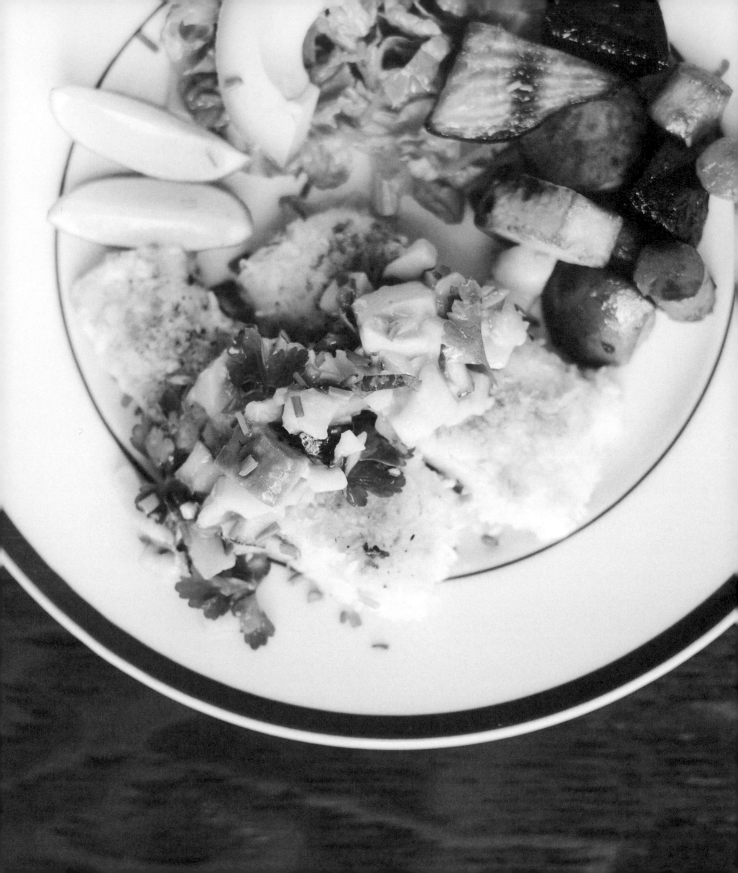

COCONUT-CRUSTED COD

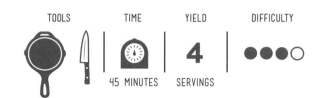

TOOLS   TIME   YIELD   DIFFICULTY

45 MINUTES   **4** SERVINGS   ●●●○

170 g coconut flour

1½ teaspoons ground ginger

¼ teaspoon sea salt

500 ml Creamy Coconut Milk
(page 46)

100 g fine shredded coconut
(unsweetened)

680 g cod fillet, skinned and
deboned and cut into 5 cm
thick strips

2 tablespoons coconut oil

Mango Salsa (page 131)

1 Combine the coconut flour, ginger and salt on a plate. Place the coconut milk in one shallow bowl and the shredded coconut in another.

2 Dip the cod strips into the coconut milk, then the coconut flour mixture, back into the coconut milk and finally back into the shredded coconut, paying special attention to coating the strips evenly.

3 Heat the coconut oil in a frying pan on high heat. Sauté the cod strips for about 5 minutes per side (depending on thickness of the fish), or until the top and bottom are nice and browned and the fish is firm.

4 Serve topped with mango salsa.

Note: Once the cod strips are in the pan, try not to fuss with them too much as the crust may crumble and fall off (most recipes for breaded fish use egg to help the dry ingredients adhere).

Storage: This dish is at its very best served immediately. You may hold it for several days in the refrigerator, but the coating will lose its crispness.

Serving Suggestions: Pomegranate and Rocket Salad with Fennel (page 146), Cabbage Slaw with Olive Avocado Dressing (page 145), Citrus-Spinach Salad (page 150), Rainbow Roasted Root Vegetables (page 188)

MEDITERRANEAN SALMON

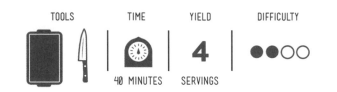

TOOLS   TIME   YIELD   DIFFICULTY

40 MINUTES   4 SERVINGS   ●●○○

1 tablespoon coconut oil

680 g wild-caught
   salmon fillet, skin on and
   deboned

95 g kalamata olives, pitted
   and minced

2–3 tablespoons chopped fresh
   flat-leaf parsley

½ lemon, juiced
   (about 1 tablespoon)

¼ teaspoon sea salt

3 tablespoons extra-virgin
   olive oil

1 Preheat the oven to 200°C.

2 Spread the coconut oil on a baking tray. Place the salmon on it, skin-side down.

3 Combine the olives, parsley, lemon juice and salt in a bowl and spread the mixture all over the fillet.

4 Bake for 15 minutes, or until the fish lightly flakes when tested with a fork. The cooking time may vary a bit depending on the thickness of the fish.

5 Drizzle with the olive oil before serving.

Storage: Keeps for a couple of days in the refrigerator.

Serving Suggestions: Parsley-Garlic Dip (page 96), Cucumber-Mint Salad (page 141), Radish and Jicama Tabbouli (page 142)

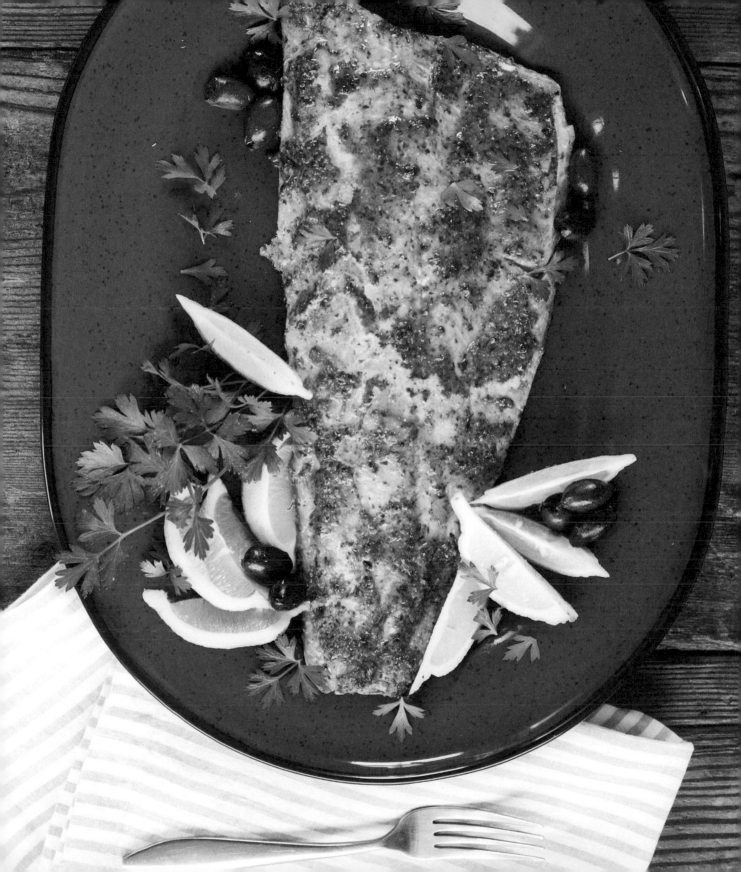

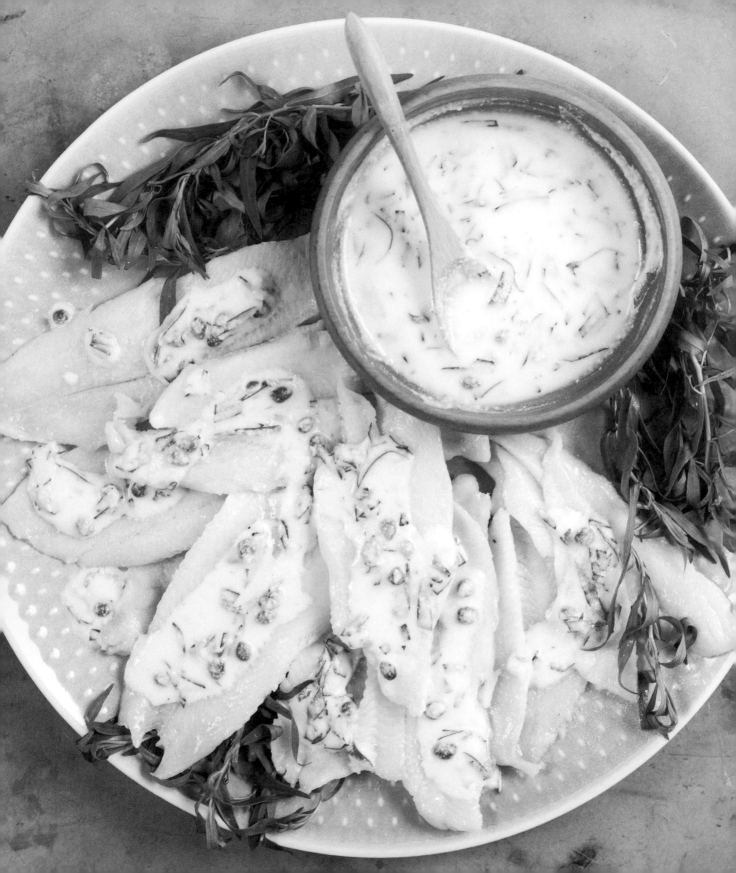

SOLE FILLET WITH TARRAGON-CAPER SAUCE

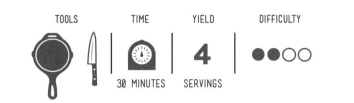

TOOLS   TIME   YIELD   DIFFICULTY

30 MINUTES   **4** SERVINGS   ●●○○

125 ml Garlic 'Mayo' (page 127)

½ lemon, juiced (about 1 tablespoon)

4 tablespoons minced tarragon

2 tablespoons capers

¼ teaspoon sea salt

2 tablespoons solid cooking fat

680 g wild-caught sole, John Dory or flounder fillets, skinned and deboned

1 Soften the mayo in a warm water bath until it is a liquid.

2 Place the mayo, lemon juice, tarragon, capers and salt in a small bowl; mix until combined. Set aside.

3 Heat the cooking fat in a frying pan on high heat. When the fat has melted and the pan is hot, sear the fish for a minute or two per side, depending on the thickness of the fillets.

4 Remove from the heat and spoon the tarragon-caper sauce over top. Serve immediately.

Storage: Keeps for a couple of days in the refrigerator.

Serving Suggestions: Market Salad (page 149), Rainbow Roasted Root Vegetables (page 188)

SEAR-ROASTED HALIBUT

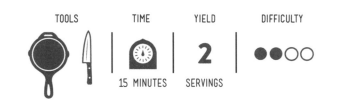

TOOLS   TIME   YIELD   DIFFICULTY

15 MINUTES   2 SERVINGS   ●●○○

½ orange, juiced
   (about 3 tablespoons)
2 tablespoons coconut aminos
½ lemon, juiced
   (about 1 tablespoon)
¼ teaspoon ground ginger
¼ teaspoon sea salt
2 tablespoons coconut flour
350 g halibut or Atlantic
   Salmon, skinned,
   deboned, and cut into
   two portions
2 tablespoons coconut oil
Fresh chives, chopped, for
   garnish

1 Preheat the oven to 200°C.

2 Combine the orange juice, coconut aminos, lemon juice, ginger and half of the salt in a small bowl; stir to combine. Place the coconut flour on a plate and set aside.

3 Sprinkle both sides of the fish with the remaining sea salt and dredge in the coconut flour, using your fingers to create a thin, even coating around all sides of the fish.

4 Heat the coconut oil in an ovenproof frying pan on high heat. When it is very hot, add the halibut and sear for 2 minutes, or until browned on the bottom. Flip the fish and place the frying pan immediately in the oven. Cook for 3 to 5 minutes, depending on the thickness of the fillets. The fish is cooked when it is no longer translucent.

5 Serve with the citrus–coconut amino sauce and garnish with the chopped chives.

Storage: Keeps for a couple of days in the refrigerator.

Serving Suggestions: Citrus-Spinach Salad (page 150), Cauliflower 'Fried Rice' (page 200), Curried Cauliflower (page 187)

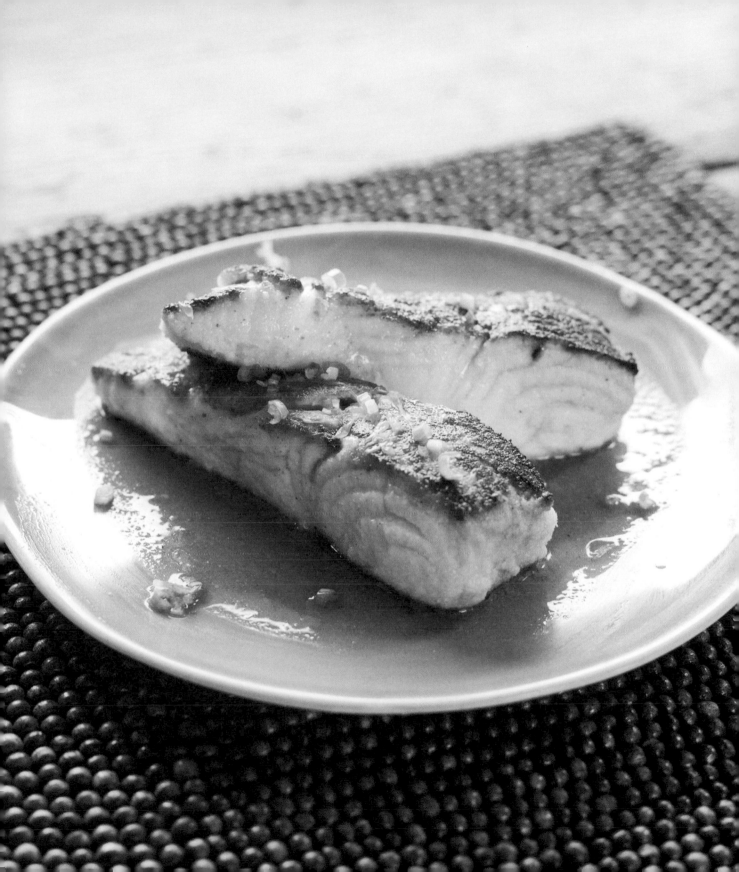

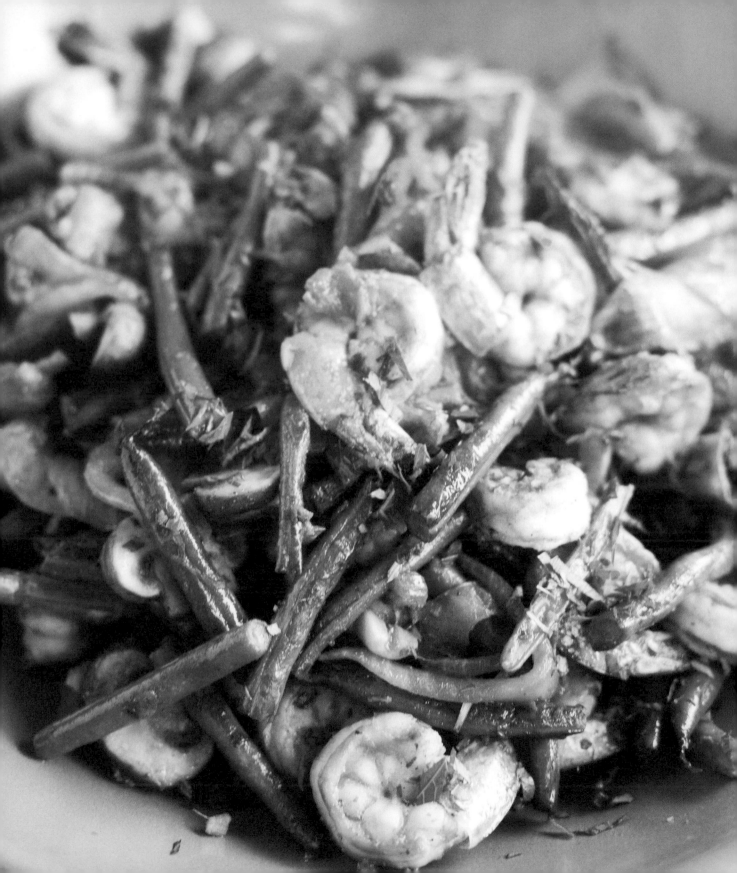

PRAWN AND
GREEN BEAN STIR-FRY

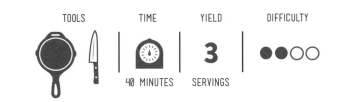

TOOLS	TIME	YIELD	DIFFICULTY
	40 MINUTES	3 SERVINGS	●●○○

2 tablespoons solid cooking fat

½ onion, halved and thinly sliced

4 cloves garlic, minced

5 cm piece ginger, peeled
  and minced

900 g green beans, trimmed
  and halved

90 g thinly sliced crimini
  mushrooms

2 tablespoons coconut aminos

1 teaspoon honey

450 g raw prawns, peeled,
  with tails left on

¼ teaspoon sea salt

Fresh flat-leaf parsley, minced,
  for garnish

1 Heat the cooking fat in a wok or large frying pan on medium–high heat. When the fat has melted and the pan is hot, add the onion and cook for 5 minutes, stirring. Add the garlic and ginger and cook, stirring for another couple of minutes. Add the green beans and cook for 10 minutes (toss and turn them so they cook evenly).

2 Add the mushrooms, coconut aminos and honey and cook for a few minutes. Add the prawns and salt and cook until the prawns are pink throughout, 3 to 4 minutes. Garnish with the parsley and serve immediately.

Storage: Keeps for a couple of days in the refrigerator.

Serving Suggestions: Cauliflower 'Fried Rice' (page 200), Curried Cauliflower (page 187), Carrot-Ginger Soup (page 162)

SALMON CHOWDER

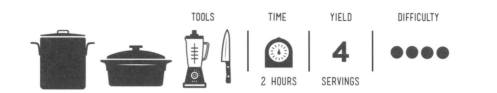

TOOLS   TIME   YIELD   DIFFICULTY

2 HOURS   **4** SERVINGS   ●●●●

Bones from 1 salmon carcass, including head and tail

1 litre water

1 bay leaf

2 tablespoons solid cooking fat

1 large onion, chopped

4 cloves garlic, minced

4 parsnips, chopped

3 carrots, chopped

2 celery stalks, chopped

1 tablespoon apple cider vinegar

1 tablespoon chopped fresh thyme

1½ teaspoons sea salt

680 g salmon fillet, skinned and deboned, cut into 4 cm chunks

250 ml Creamy Coconut Milk (page 46)

½ lemon, juiced (about 1 tablespoon)

3 spring onions, thinly sliced

1 To make the broth, place the salmon carcass, water and bay leaf in a stockpot, bring to a boil, cover, and turn down to a bare simmer for 45 minutes. It is essential to cook this at the lowest simmer possible.

2 Remove and discard the carcass and bay leaf. Strain the broth through a fine sieve into a large bowl and set it aside.

3 Heat the cooking fat in a heavy-bottomed pot on medium heat. When the fat has melted and the pan is hot, add the onion and cook for 5 minutes, stirring. Add the garlic and cook for another couple of minutes, until fragrant. Add the parsnips, carrots and celery; cook another 5 minutes, stirring, until the vegetables are lightly browned.

4 Add the reserved fish broth, vinegar, thyme and salt to the pot and bring to a boil. Cover and turn down to a bare simmer, and cook for 30 minutes or until the vegetables are tender.

5 Place 500 ml of the soup in a blender, leaving the carrots behind, if possible, so as not to turn the soup orange. Blend until smooth, then add the purée back to the soup.

6 Add the salmon chunks and coconut milk to the soup and cook for a few minutes, just until the soup is piping hot (do not let the soup boil).

7 Add the lemon juice and serve garnished with spring onions.

Note: Tastes best served fresh, but if you must reheat, do so gently over low heat.

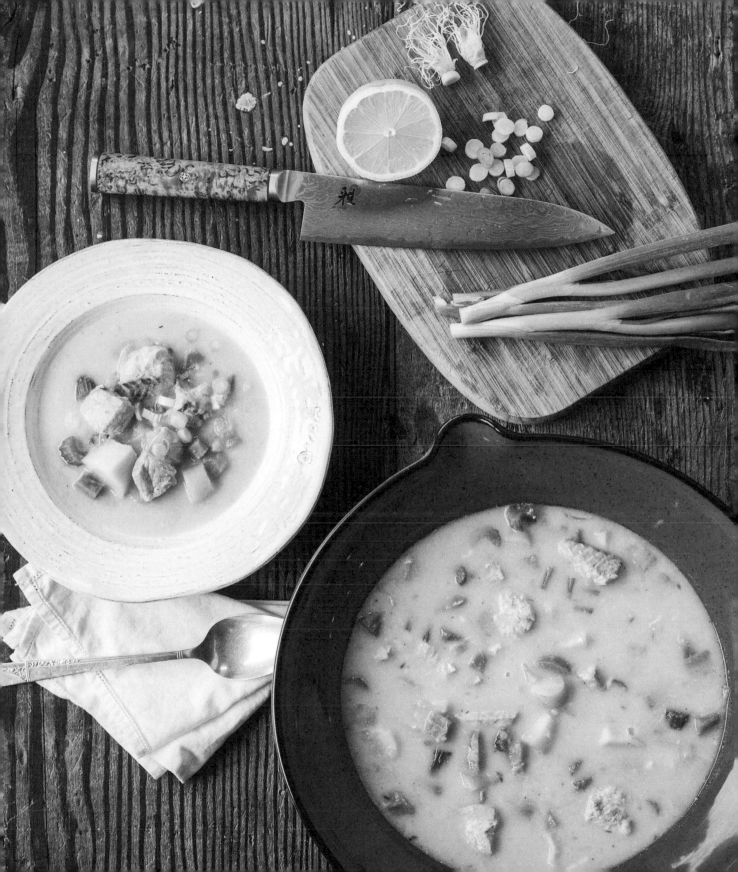

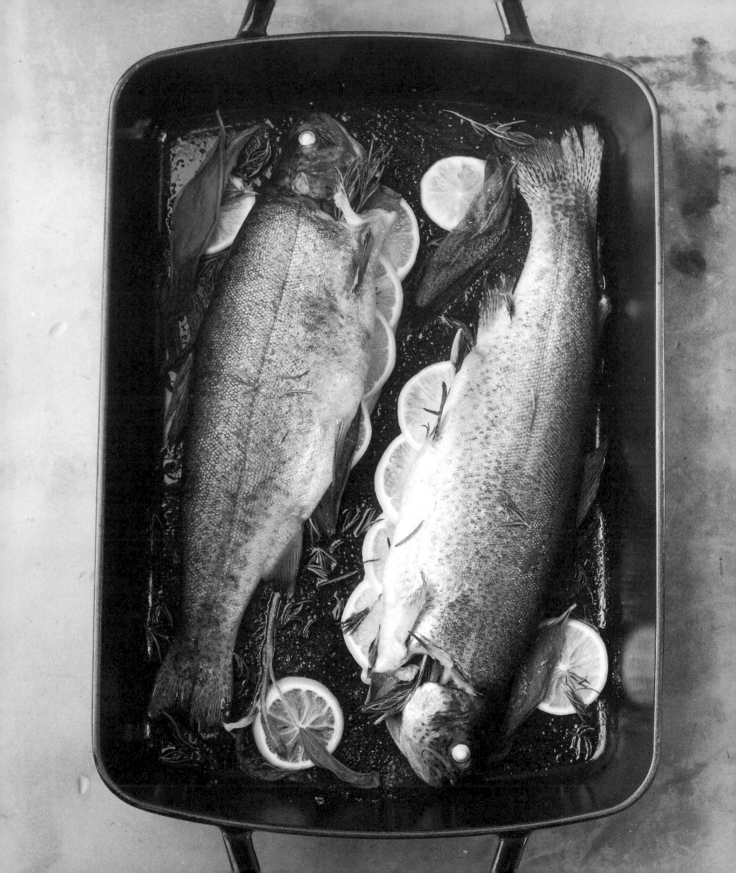

HERB-STUFFED TROUT

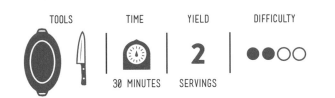

TOOLS   TIME   YIELD   DIFFICULTY

30 MINUTES   **2** SERVINGS   ●●○○

1 tablespoon solid cooking fat

2 whole trout (about 450 g each), scaled and gutted

½ teaspoon sea salt

1 lemon, sliced into thin rounds

4 sprigs of fresh rosemary

4 sprigs of fresh thyme

You will need:

Kitchen twine

1 Preheat the oven to 230°C.

2 Coat the bottom of a baking dish with the cooking fat. Sprinkle the salt all over the inside and outside of the fish, and place them in the dish.

3 Fill the cavity of each fish with a few lemon slices and a couple large sprigs of the herbs. Using the twine, tie a loop around the middle of each fish so that the contents stay inside. Alternatively, pin the thinnest part of each belly closed, using skewers or toothpicks.

4 Roast for 15 minutes, or until the flesh flakes easily when tested with a fork.

5 Serve whole, eating around the bones, herbs and lemon in the cavity.

Note: If you have someone in your family who is a fisherman/woman, wild trout is much preferred over the commercial farmed variety!

Serving Suggestions: Emerald Kale Salad (page 138), Cinnamon-Scented Butternut Squash (page 184), Puréed Parsnips (page 196), Carrot-Ginger Soup (page 162)

CLAM CHOWDER

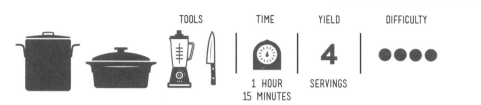

TOOLS

TIME
1 HOUR
15 MINUTES

YIELD
4
SERVINGS

DIFFICULTY
●●●●

1 tablespoon sea salt

1.3 kg clams

375 ml filtered water

4 rashers sugar-free bacon

1 small onion, chopped

2 carrots, chopped

5 cloves garlic, minced

1 tablespoon fresh thyme

1 bay leaf

900 g celeriac, peeled and cut into small cubes

250 ml Creamy Coconut Milk (page 46)

3 spring onions, sliced thinly, for garnish

1 Add the salt to a bowl of cool water and stir to dissolve. Add the clams and allow them to soak for 20 minutes.

2 Clean the clam shells thoroughly with a wire brush or a stiff vegetable brush, discarding any that are broken.

3 Bring the filtered water to a boil in a large pot. Add the clams, cover and reduce the heat to a simmer. After about 4 minutes the clams should start opening; once they do, pull them out one-by-one. Continue doing this until all the clams have cooked, about another 4 minutes. If there are any that haven't opened at this point, throw them away. Set the clams aside to cool, then strain the clam broth, reserving 375 ml for the soup.

4 In a heavy-bottomed pot, cook the bacon rashers until they are crispy, turning as needed. Remove them from the pot, leaving the fat. Add the onion and cook for 5 minutes, then add the carrots, garlic, thyme and bay leaf and cook, stirring, for 5 more minutes. Add the reserved clam broth and the celeriac, bring to a boil, then cover and simmer for 5 to 10 minutes, or until the celeriac is soft.

5 Remove the clams from their shells and chop the bacon into bits. Set aside.

6 When the celeriac has finished cooking, turn off the heat, remove the bay leaf and transfer half of the mixture to a blender. Blend until very smooth, then add the purée back to the pot.

7 Stir in the coconut milk, clams and bacon bits. Garnish with chopped spring onions.

Note: Tastes best served fresh, but if you must reheat, do so gently over low heat.

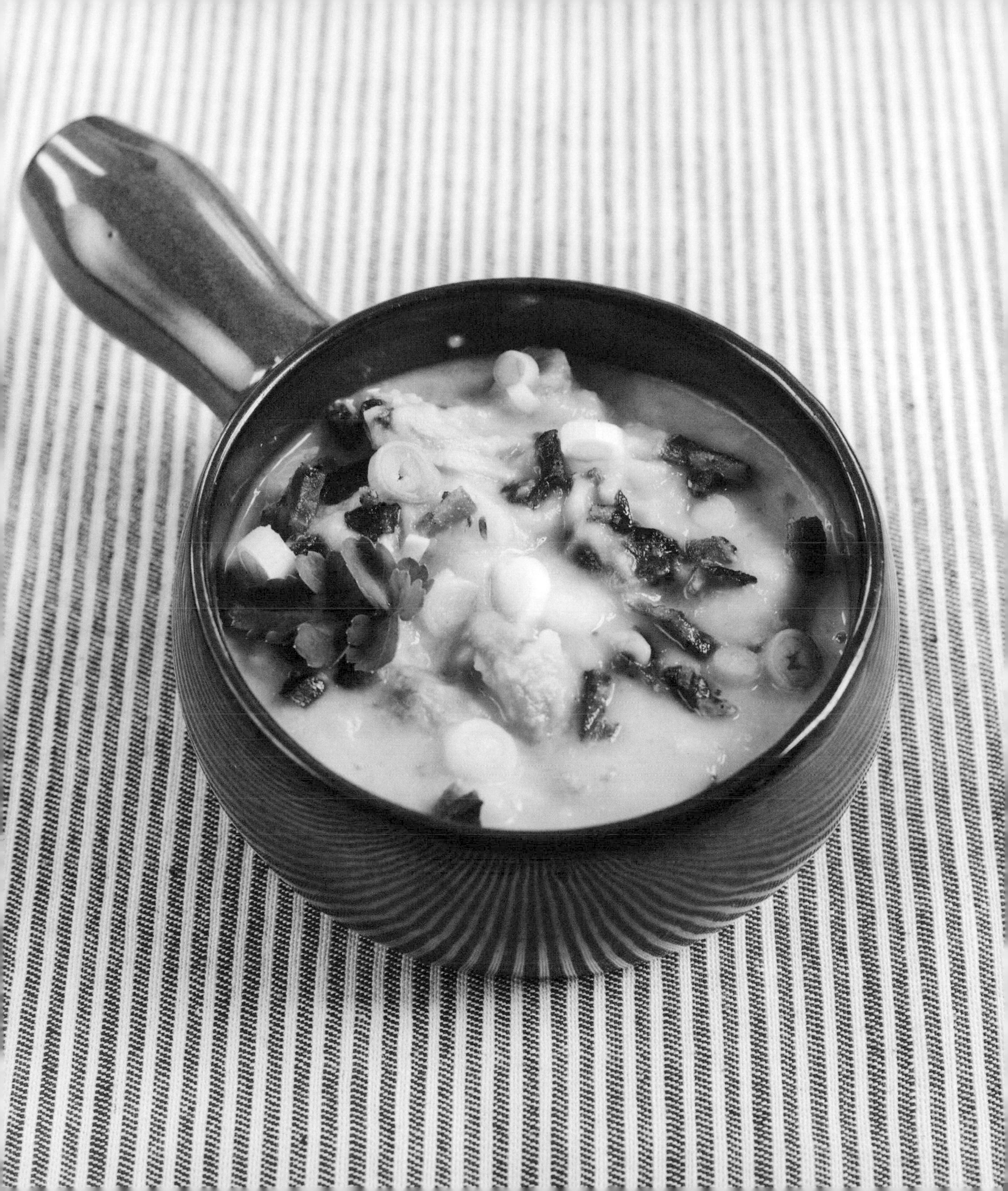

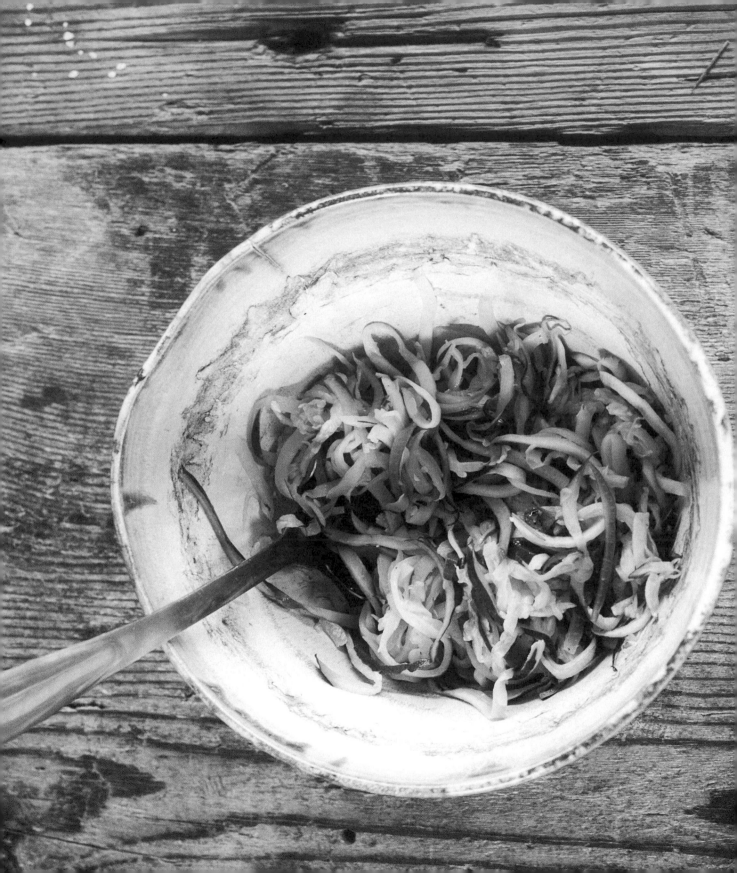

BEEF + LAMB

CRANBERRY-BRAISED SHORT RIBS

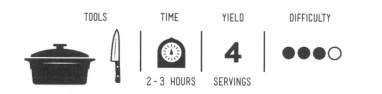

TOOLS	TIME	YIELD	DIFFICULTY
	2 - 3 HOURS	4 SERVINGS	●●●○

1 tablespoon solid cooking fat

1.8 kg grass-fed beef short ribs

250 ml Bone Broth (page 34)

250 ml unsweetened cranberry juice

90 g fresh or frozen cranberries

1 tablespoon apple cider vinegar

1 bay leaf

¼ teaspoon sea salt

2 tablespoons chopped fresh flat-leaf parsley

1 Preheat the oven to 150°C.

2 Heat the fat in a large, heavy-bottomed ovenproof pot with a lid on medium–high heat. Working in batches, brown the ribs well on all sides.

3 Add the bone broth, cranberry juice, cranberries, vinegar, bay leaf and salt to the pot. The liquid should come up to about one-third of the level of the meat—if any less, add a little bit more broth or water.

4 Making sure that your lid fits tightly, braise for 2 to 3 hours in the oven, checking periodically that the liquid is barely simmering, and that there is enough liquid (you shouldn't have a problem if the lid seals well). It is finished when the meat is falling off the bone.

5 Carefully transfer the short ribs to a plate and cover the meat. Strain the liquid into a large bowl, then pour it into a saucepan, bring it to a boil, and reduce the quantity by about half (you should have about 185 ml).

6 Serve with some of the cooking juices poured over the ribs and the parsley sprinkled on top.

Storage: Keeps in the refrigerator for several days.

Serving Suggestions: Puréed Parsnips (page 196), Mashed Sweet Potatoes (page 192), Sautéed Market Greens (page 183), Rosemary Grilled Asparagus (page 195)

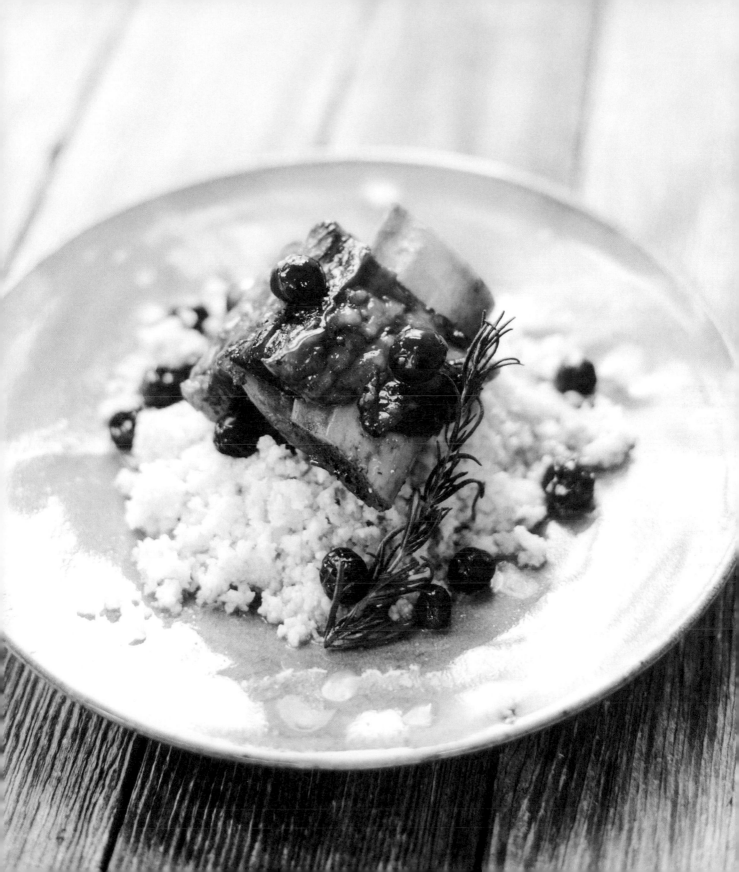

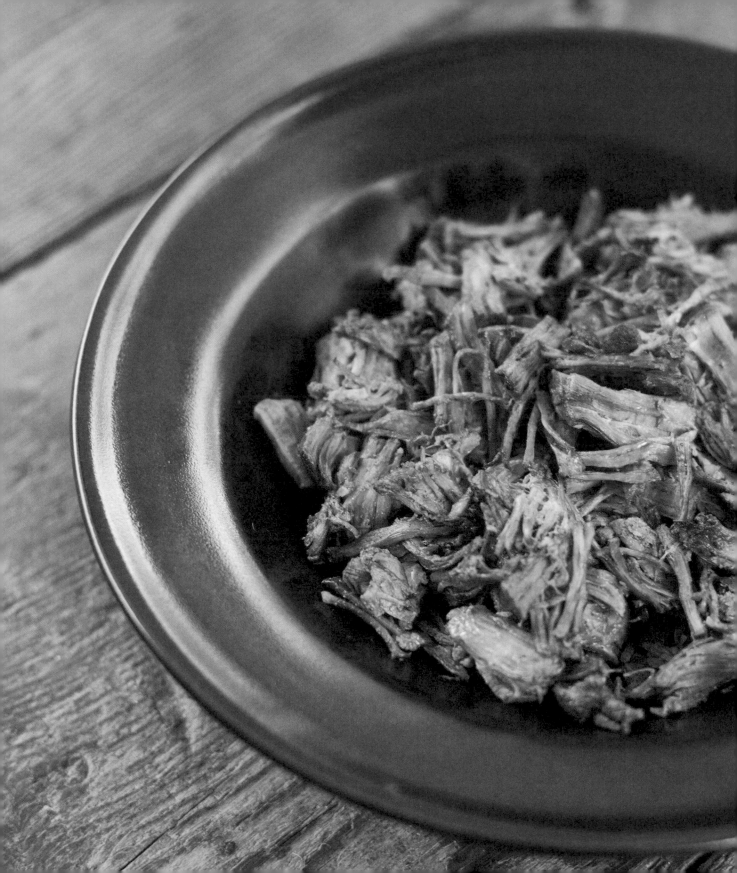

SHREDDED ROAST BEEF

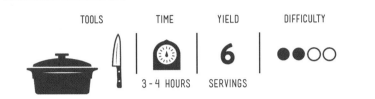

TOOLS   TIME   YIELD   DIFFICULTY

6

3 - 4 HOURS   SERVINGS

1 tablespoon solid cooking fat

Sea salt

1 x 1.3–1.8 kg beef brisket,
cut into 2 or 3 big chunks

375 ml Bone Broth (page 34)

1 tablespoon apple cider vinegar

A large handful of fresh herbs
(thyme, rosemary, sage and
oregano all work great)

1 Preheat the oven to 140°C.

2 Generously apply salt to the meat.

3 Heat the cooking fat in an ovenproof pot with a lid on medium–high heat. When the fat has melted and the pan is hot, brown the chunks of beef on all sides. Turn off the heat.

4 Add the bone broth and vinegar to the pot along with the fresh herbs. Ensuring that your lid is on tightly, cook for 3 to 4 hours, checking periodically to make sure there is liquid in the bottom of the pot. The meat is finished cooking when it pulls apart easily with a fork.

5 Remove the meat from the pot and let it cool for a couple of minutes. Meanwhile, pass the juices from the pot through a sieve, pour it into a small saucepan, and bring it to a simmer. Reduce the liquid until the quantity is about 185 ml (about 15 minutes).

6 Once the meat has cooled a little bit, shred it into bits using two forks or your hands.

7 Add the reduced pan juices back to the shredded beef and combine.

Storage: Keeps in the refrigerator for several days. Also freezes well.

Serving Suggestions: Serve on lettuce boats or as a salad with Mango Salsa (page 131) and Guacamole (page 128).

THREE-HERB BEEF PATTIES

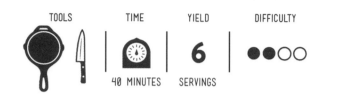

TOOLS | TIME | YIELD | DIFFICULTY

40 MINUTES | **6** SERVINGS | ●●○○

900 g grass-fed beef mince
1 tablespoon finely chopped
fresh rosemary
1 tablespoon finely chopped
fresh thyme
1 tablespoon finely chopped
fresh sage
1 teaspoon sea salt
1 tablespoon solid cooking fat

1 In a large bowl, combine the beef mince, fresh herbs and salt.

2 Using your hands, form into 12 patties.

3 Heat the cooking fat in a cast-iron frying pan on medium heat. Cook the patties for about 5 to 8 minutes per side, until nicely browned on the outside and cooked throughout. Alternatively, bake the patties in the oven for about 20 minutes at 200°C.

Storage: Keeps in the refrigerator for several days. Also freezes well.

Variation: Make meatballs and serve with cooked spaghetti squash or courgette (zucchini) noodles and Coconut-Basil Pesto (page 124) or Nomato Sauce (page 135).

Serving Suggestions: Emerald Kale Salad (page 138), Market Salad (page 149)

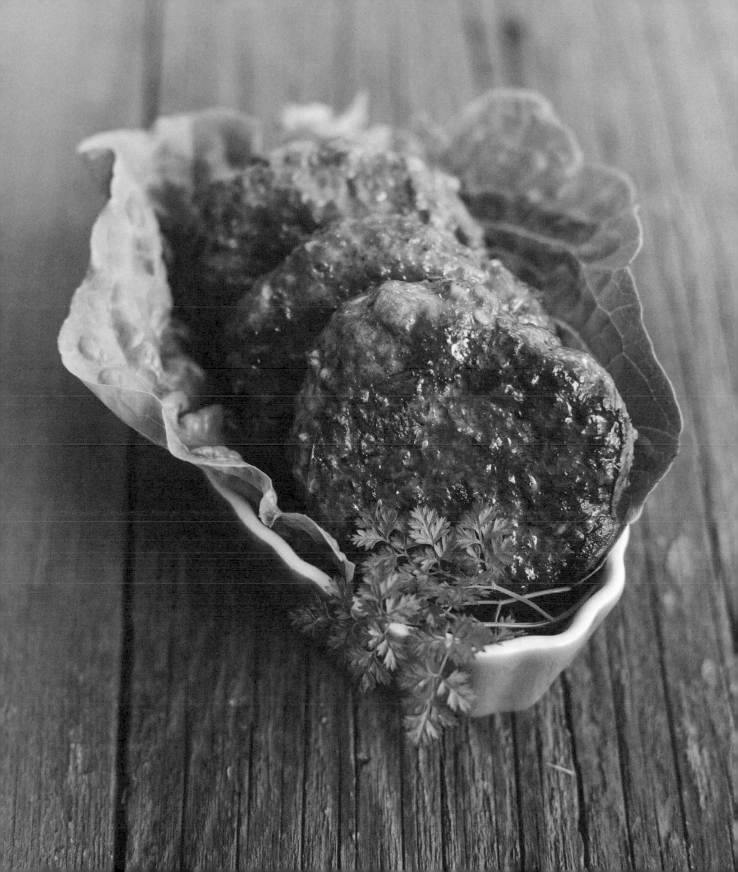

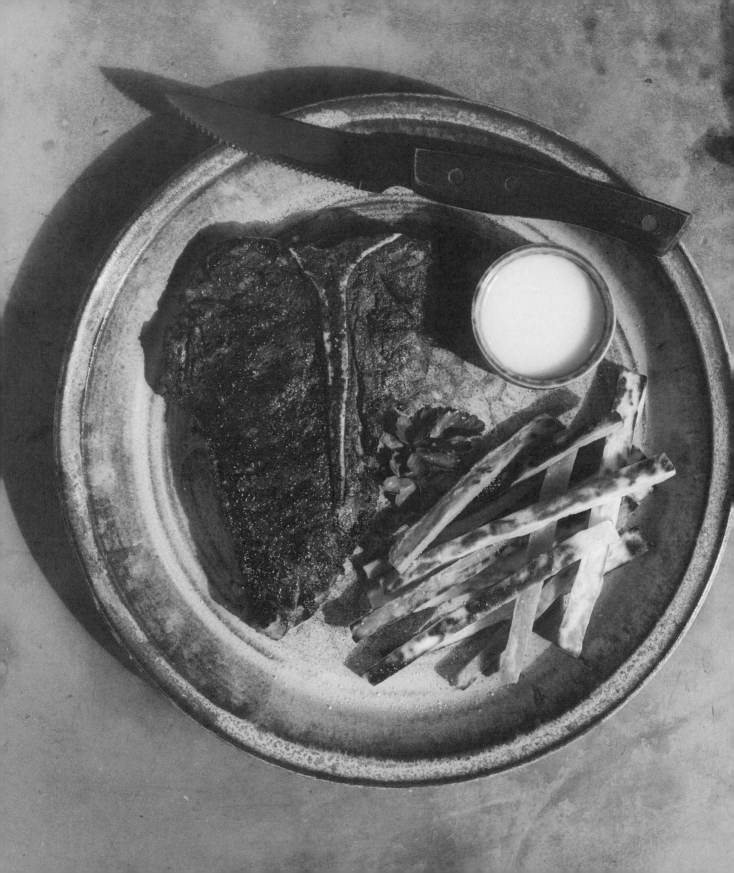

DRY-RUBBED STEAK

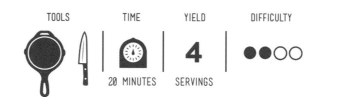

TOOLS	TIME	YIELD	DIFFICULTY
	20 MINUTES	**4** SERVINGS	●●○○

900 g grass-fed beef steaks
(such as T-Bone)
1 tablespoon coconut oil

Cinnamon-Sage Variation:
1½ tablespoons sea salt
¾ tablespoon dried sage
¾ teaspoon ground cinnamon

Herbed Variation:
1 tablespoon smoked sea salt
1 tablespoon dried rosemary
1 tablespoon dried thyme
½ tablespoon dried sage

1 Choose which variation of the rub you will be making, and combine the salt, herbs and spices together in a small bowl.

2 Rub the mixture on both sides of the steaks.

3 Heat the coconut oil in a cast-iron frying pan on medium–high heat. When the fat has melted and the pan is hot, cook the steaks 5 to 7 minutes per side, or until desired doneness is reached.

Note: This recipe also works fantastically on the barbecue.

Variation: Try using lamb chops or steaks instead of beef.

Serving Suggestions: Root Vegetable Chips (page 95), Cabbage Slaw with Olive-Avocado Dressing (page 145), Market Salad (page 149), Rosemary Grilled Asparagus (page 195), Sweet Potato Chips with Garlic 'Mayo' (page 209)

CITRUS-THYME POT ROAST

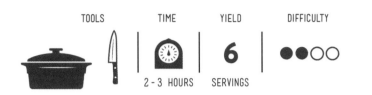

TOOLS | TIME | YIELD | DIFFICULTY

2 - 3 HOURS | SERVINGS

6

●●○○

1 tablespoon solid cooking fat

900–1.3 kg grass-fed
beef braising joint (such as
rump, blade or brisket)

185 ml Bone Broth (page 34)

2 tablespoons apple cider vinegar

1 orange, juiced (about 80 ml)

1 bay leaf

1½ teaspoons sea salt

3 carrots, cut into 5 cm chunks

2 parsnips, peeled and cut into
5 cm chunks

2 tablespoons chopped
fresh thyme

1 Preheat the oven to 150°C.

2 Heat the cooking fat in the bottom of an ovenproof pot with a lid on medium–high heat. Brown the meat well on all sides and remove it from the pot.

3 Add the bone broth, cider vinegar, orange juice, bay leaf and salt to the pot and stir to combine.

4 Place the roast in the pot and surround it with the carrots and parsnips. Sprinkle the thyme all over the meat and the vegetables.

5 Making sure the lid fits properly, cover the pot and braise the meat for 2 to 3 hours in the oven, checking periodically to make sure that it is covered by at least a third of liquid (you shouldn't have a problem if the lid seals well). It is finished when the meat is easily pulled apart with a fork.

6 Remove the bay leaf and serve the meat and vegetables with some of the cooking juices.

Variation: Feel free to use cranberry juice instead of orange, or rosemary or sage instead of the thyme.

Storage: Keeps in the refrigerator for several days.

Serving Suggestions: Citrus-Spinach Salad (page 150), Cinnamon-Scented Butternut Squash (page 184), Puréed Parsnips (page 196), Roasted Mixed Vegetables (page 199), Sautéed Market Greens (page 183)

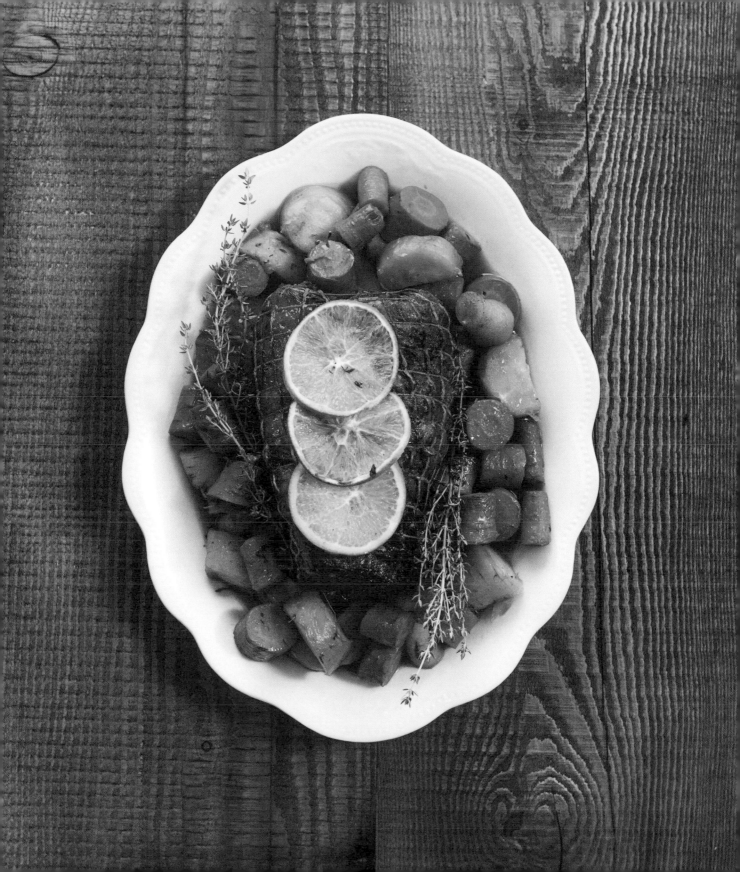

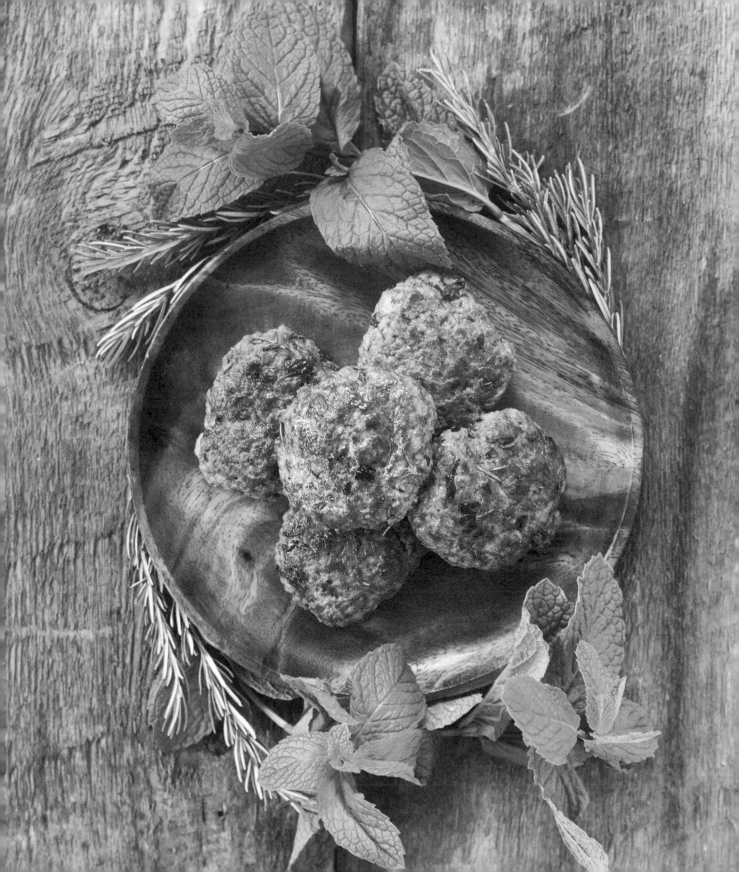

ROSEMARY-MINT LAMB PATTIES

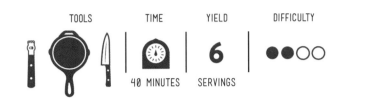

TOOLS	TIME	YIELD	DIFFICULTY
	40 MINUTES	**6** SERVINGS	●●○○

900 g lamb mince

2 tablespoons finely chopped fresh mint

1 tablespoon finely chopped fresh rosemary

1 teaspoon sea salt

½ teaspoon lemon zest

1 tablespoon solid cooking fat

1 In a large bowl, combine the lamb, mint, rosemary, salt and lemon zest.

2 Using your hands, form into 12 patties.

3 Heat some of the cooking fat in a cast-iron frying pan on medium heat. Cook the patties for 5 to 8 minutes per side, until nicely browned on the outside and cooked throughout. Alternatively, bake the patties in the oven for about 20 minutes at 200°C.

Storage: Keeps in the refrigerator for several days. Also freezes well.

Serving Suggestions: Cucumber-Mint Salad (page 141), Radish and Jicama Tabbouli (page 142), Emerald Kale Salad (page 138)

GARLIC BEEF AND BROCCOLI

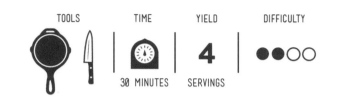

TOOLS

TIME
30 MINUTES

YIELD
4
SERVINGS

DIFFICULTY
●●○○

½ tablespoon solid cooking fat

900 g grass-fed beef steaks, cut into 5 mm thick slices

5 cloves garlic, minced

4 cm piece ginger, peeled and minced

1 bunch broccoli, chopped

2 tablespoons water or Bone Broth (page 34)

125 ml coconut aminos

½ lemon, juiced (about 1 tablespoon)

¼ teaspoon sea salt

1 Heat the cooking fat in a wok or large frying pan on medium-high heat.

2 When the fat has melted and the pan is hot, sauté the steak slices, stirring, for 5 to 7 minutes. Remove and set aside.

3 Lower the heat to medium and add the garlic and ginger, stirring and cooking until fragrant, about 1 minute. Add the broccoli and cook for a few minutes, until lightly browned. Add the water, cover and reduce the heat to medium-low. Cook for about 10 minutes, stirring occasionally, until the broccoli is tender.

4 Add the coconut aminos, lemon juice, salt and beef slices back to the pan and sauté, tossing to combine, for a minute or two. Serve immediately.

Storage: Keeps in the refrigerator for several days.

Serving Suggestions: Cauliflower 'Fried Rice' (page 200), Curried Cauliflower (page 187)

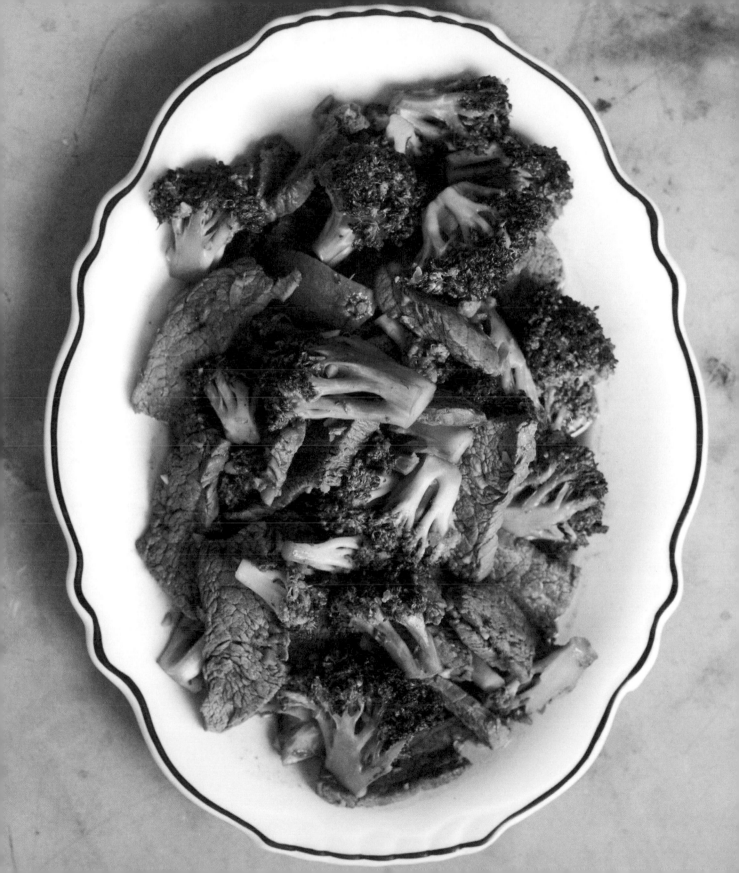

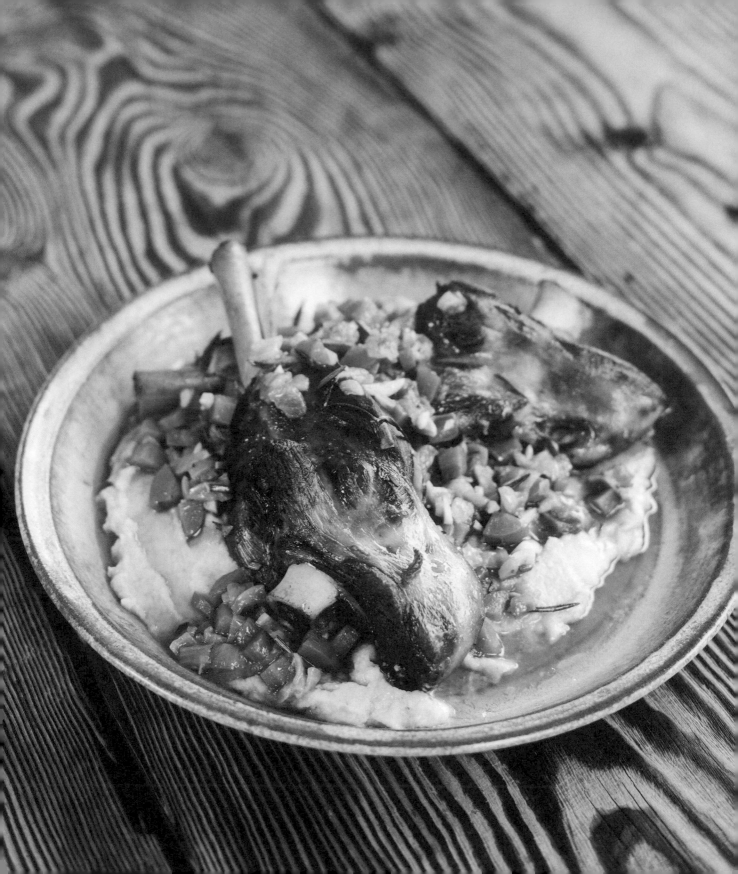

BRAISED LAMB SHANKS
WITH PARSNIP PURÉE

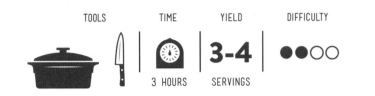

TOOLS	TIME	YIELD	DIFFICULTY
	3 HOURS	**3-4** SERVINGS	●●○○

2 tablespoons solid cooking fat

1.3–1.8 kg lamb shanks

1 onion, finely chopped

2 carrots, finely chopped

5 cloves garlic, minced

3 tablespoons minced fresh
   rosemary

1 tablespoon apple cider vinegar

375 ml Bone Broth (page 34)

¼ teaspoon sea salt

1 recipe Parsnip Purée (page 196)

Fresh flat-leaf parsley, chopped,
   for garnish

1 Preheat the oven to 150°C.

2 Heat the cooking fat in a large ovenproof pot with a lid on a medium heat. When the fat has melted and the pan is hot, brown the lamb shanks well on all sides, about 8 minutes. Remove from the pot and set aside.

3 Add the onion, carrots, garlic and rosemary; cook for 5 to 7 minutes, stirring, until lightly browned.

4 Turn off the heat, add the vinegar, bone broth, salt and return the shanks to the pot. The liquid should come up one-third to one-half the level of the shanks. If it is too low, add a little more water or broth. Cover with a tight-fitting lid and cook in the oven for 2 to 3 hours, until the meat is falling off the bone. Take the lid off the pot for the last 20 minutes of cooking.

5 Serve on a bed of puréed parsnips with some of the pan juices drizzled on top. Garnish with the parsley.

Variation: Serve on a bed of Mashed Sweet Potatoes (page 192) instead of the parsnips, if you like.

Storage: Keeps in the refrigerator for several days.

Serving Suggestions: Sautéed Market Greens (page 183), Brussels Sprouts with Crispy Bacon (page 191), Rosemary Grilled Asparagus (page 195)

PORTOBELLO 'BURGER'

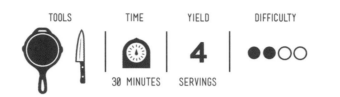

TOOLS | TIME | YIELD | DIFFICULTY

30 MINUTES | **4 SERVINGS** | ●●○○

4 tablespoons Garlic 'Mayo'
(page 127)

2 tablespoons solid cooking fat,
melted

4 portobello mushrooms,
brushed clean and stalks
removed

½ onion, sliced into
thick rings

Sea salt

4 to 8 leaves soft lettuce
(not romaine)

4 Three-Herb Beef Patties
(page 262), cooked and kept
warm

1 avocado, peeled, destoned
and sliced

1 Soften the mayo in a warm water bath until it is a liquid.

2 Heat half the cooking fat in a frying pan or griddle pan over medium heat.

3 Brush the rest of the fat on the portobello caps and onion, also sprinkling with sea salt. Add the mushrooms and onions to the pan and cook for 10 to 15 minutes, flipping once, until fully cooked. Turn off the heat and set aside to cool for a few minutes.

4 Grab a leaf or two of lettuce and construct a 'burger' using a beef patty, a tablespoon of mayo, some onion rings and a portobello. Finish with several slices of avocado.

Serving Suggestions: Rainbow Root Vegetable Chips (page 95), Sweet Potato Chips (page 207) and Garlic 'Mayo' (page 127)

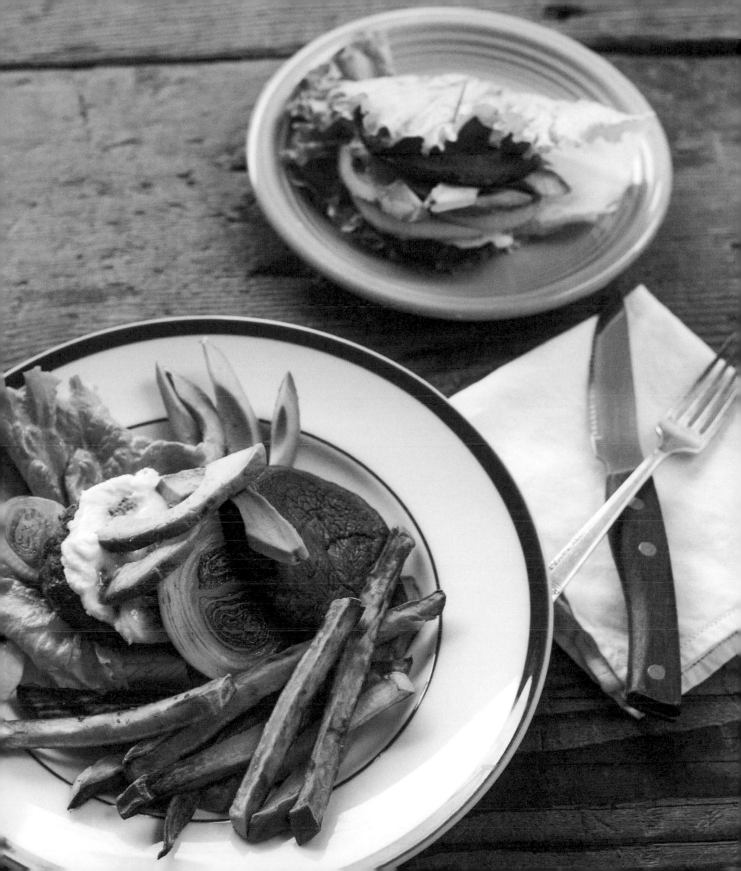

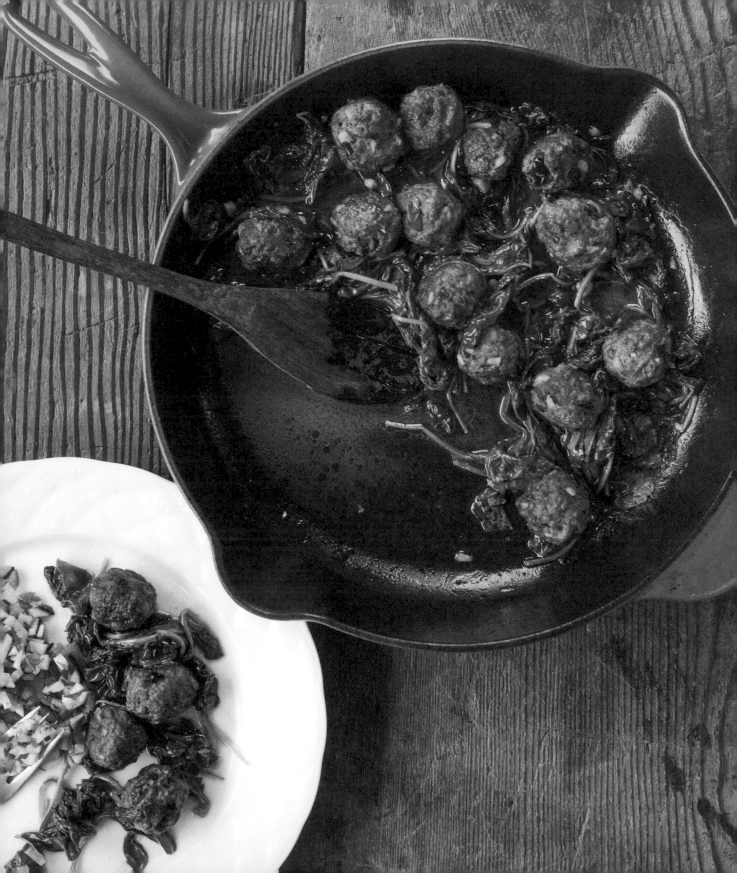

LAMB MEATBALLS WITH GARLIC AND SPINACH

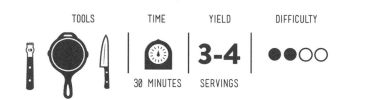

TOOLS   TIME   YIELD   DIFFICULTY

3-4

30 MINUTES   SERVINGS

6 kalamata olives, minced

3 cloves garlic, minced

½ teaspoon lemon zest

½ teaspoon ground cinnamon

½ teaspoon sea salt

450 g lamb mince

2 tablespoons solid cooking fat

125 ml Bone Broth (page 34)

180 g baby spinach leaves

½ lemon, juiced
  (about 1 tablespoon)

1 Combine the olives, garlic, lemon zest, cinnamon and salt in a bowl.

2 Add the lamb, mix thoroughly, and form into 2.5 cm meatballs.

3 Heat the cooking fat in a frying pan on medium–high heat.

4 When the fat has melted and the pan is hot, cook the meatballs for 5 minutes, turning periodically to brown evenly. Add the bone broth and cover, cooking for another 5 to 6 minutes until the meatballs are cooked throughout. Turn off the heat, add the spinach and stir until wilted.

5 Drizzle with lemon juice and serve.

Storage: Keeps in the refrigerator for several days.

Serving Suggestions: Puréed Parsnips (page 196), Mashed Sweet Potatoes (page 192)

ROSEMARY SHREDDED BEEF

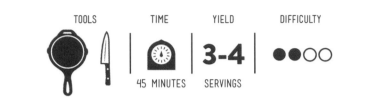

TOOLS | TIME | YIELD | DIFFICULTY

45 MINUTES | **3-4** SERVINGS | ●●○○

3 tablespoons solid cooking fat

3 medium sweet potatoes, peeled and chopped into 2.5 cm cubes

½ onion, chopped

170 g chopped courgette (zucchini)

4 cloves garlic, minced

2 tablespoons minced fresh rosemary

½ teaspoon sea salt

200 g Shredded Roast Beef (page 261)

1 Heat 2 tablespoons of the cooking fat in the bottom of a large cast-iron pan or frying pan on medium heat.

2 When the fat has melted and the pan is hot, add the sweet potatoes and cook, stirring, for 10 minutes, or until they are slightly soft, but not all the way cooked. Add the onion and cook for another 5 minutes, then add the courgette, garlic, rosemary and salt, stirring. Cook for 10 more minutes.

3 Add the shredded beef and the rest of the cooking fat. Cook for another few minutes, or until the beef is heated through and all of the vegetables are soft.

Variation: Try using hard winter squash (like butternut or acorn) instead of the sweet potato.

Storage: Keeps in the refrigerator for several days.

Serving Suggestions: Sautéed Market Greens (page 183), Seared Broccolini with Coconut-Basil Pesto (page 204)

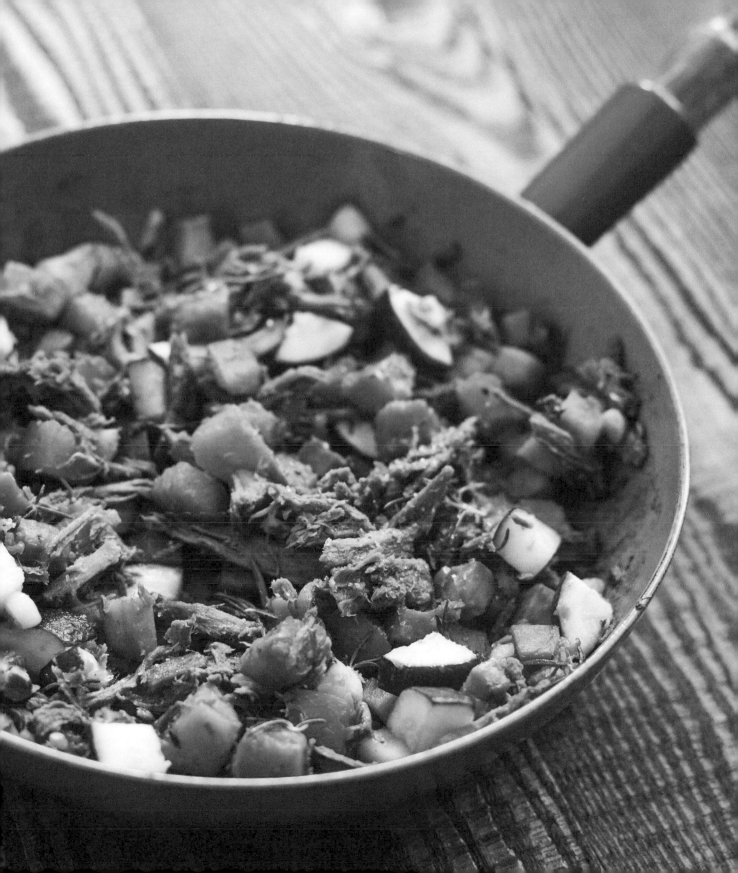

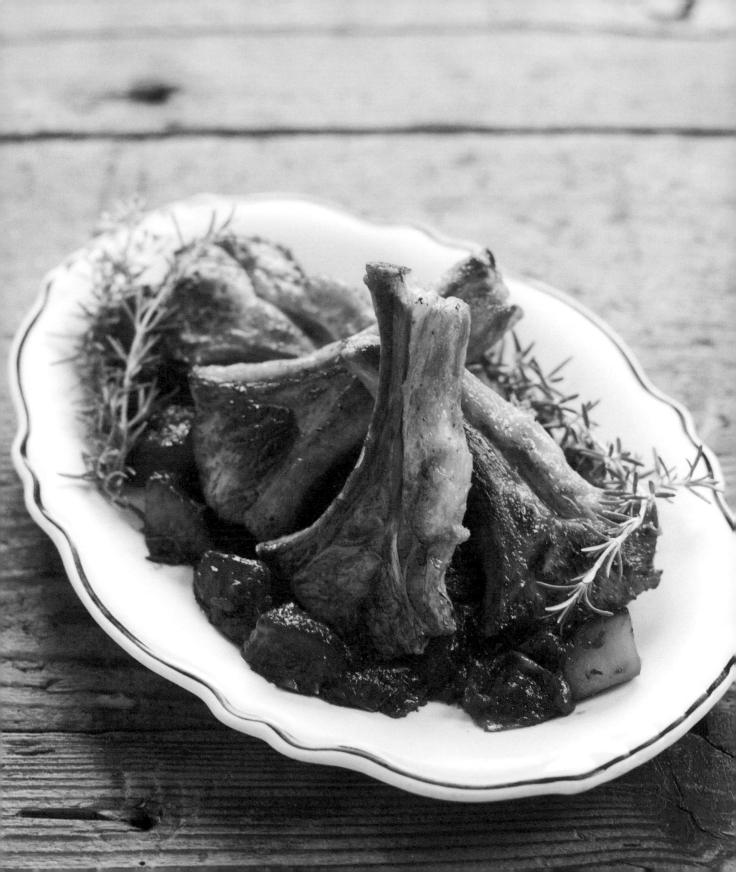

LAMB CHOPS WITH ROSEMARY-PLUM SAUCE

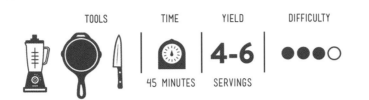

TOOLS	TIME	YIELD	DIFFICULTY
	45 MINUTES	**4-6** SERVINGS	●●●○

2 tablespoons solid cooking fat

½ onion, chopped

2 cloves garlic, minced

3 firm plums, chopped into 5 cm pieces, kept separate

1 tablespoon minced rosemary

¼ teaspoon sea salt

900 g lamb chops

1 Heat 1 tablespoon of the cooking fat in a saucepan on medium heat. When the fat has melted and the pan is hot, add the onion and cook for about 5 minutes. Add the garlic and cook for another minute, stirring. Add 1 of the chopped plums and cook for about 10 minutes, stirring, until soft. Turn off the heat.

2 Transfer the mixture to a blender and purée it. Add the mixture back to the pan, along with the remaining chopped plums, rosemary and half of the salt. Turn the heat to medium and cook for 10 more minutes, or until the sauce has thickened and the plums are soft.

3 Sprinkle the remaining salt on the lamb chops, and heat the remaining cooking fat in a frying pan on high heat. Sauté the lamb chops for 5 to 8 minutes per side, or until desired doneness is reached.

4 Serve the chops with plum sauce drizzled over the top.

Storage: Keeps in the refrigerator for several days.

Serving Suggestions: Cucumber-Mint Salad (page 141), Radish and Jicama Tabbouli (page 142), Puréed Parsnips (page 196)

'SPAGHETTI' AND MEATBALLS

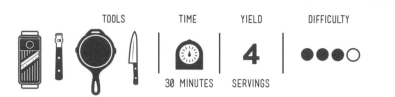

TOOLS | **TIME** 30 MINUTES | **YIELD** 4 SERVINGS | **DIFFICULTY** ●●●○

900 g grass-fed beef mince
1 tablespoon minced fresh
  rosemary
1 tablespoon minced fresh thyme
1 tablespoon minced fresh sage
1 teaspoon sea salt
2 tablespoons solid cooking fat
1 recipe Nomato Sauce
  (page 135)
4 courgettes (zucchini), cut
  into noodles with a mandoline
  or spiralizer
Fresh basil, for garnish
Zest of 1 lemon, for garnish

1 In a large bowl, combine the beef mince, fresh herbs and salt.

2 Using your hands, form into large, 5–7.5 cm meatballs.

3 Heat 1 tablespoon of the cooking fat in a frying pan on medium heat. Add the meatballs and brown well on all sides. Add the Nomato Sauce, cover and turn down to a simmer. Cook for another 10 to 15 minutes, or until the meatballs are cooked throughout.

4 Meanwhile, heat the remaining cooking fat in the bottom of another frying pan or a wok. When the fat has melted and the pan is hot, add the courgette noodles and cook, tossing them gently, until they soften (about 5 minutes).

5 Serve a plate of courgette noodles, meatballs and sauce garnished with the chopped basil and lemon zest.

Variation: Feel free to use any kind of minced meat for this recipe, or a combination. You can also replace the courgette noodles with cooked spaghetti squash.

Storage: Keeps in the refrigerator for several days.

Serving Suggestions: Emerald Kale Salad (page 138), Brussels Sprouts with Crispy Bacon (page 191), Sautéed Market Greens (page 183)

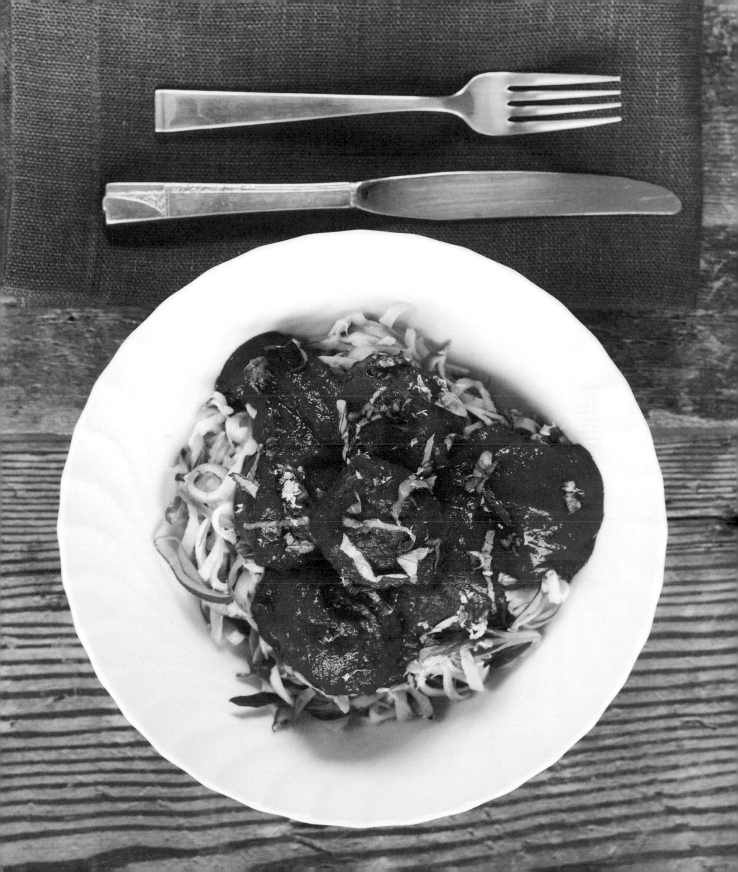

SWEET TREATS

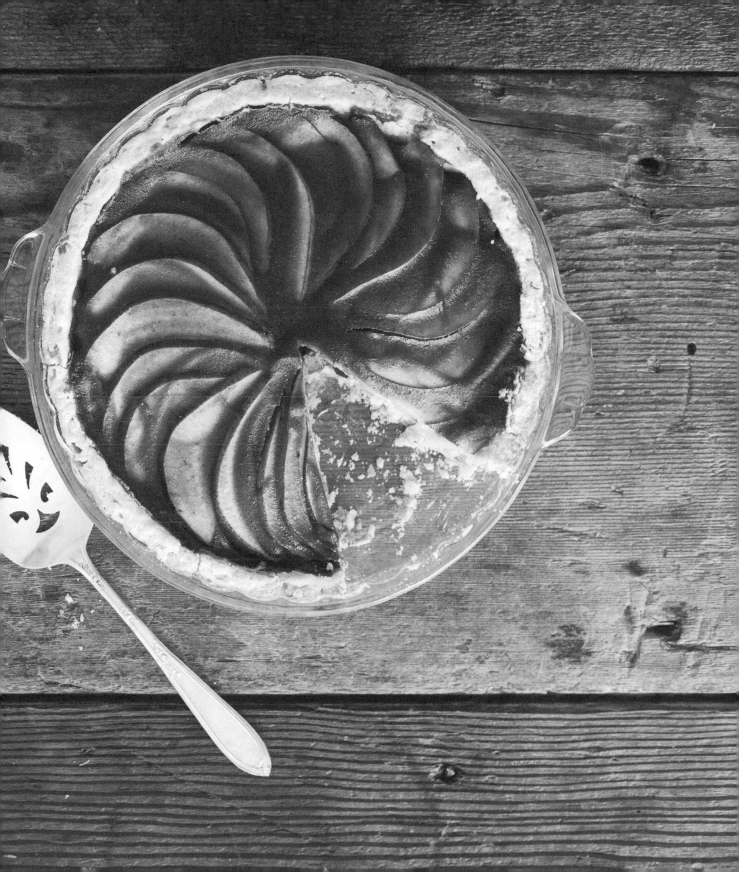

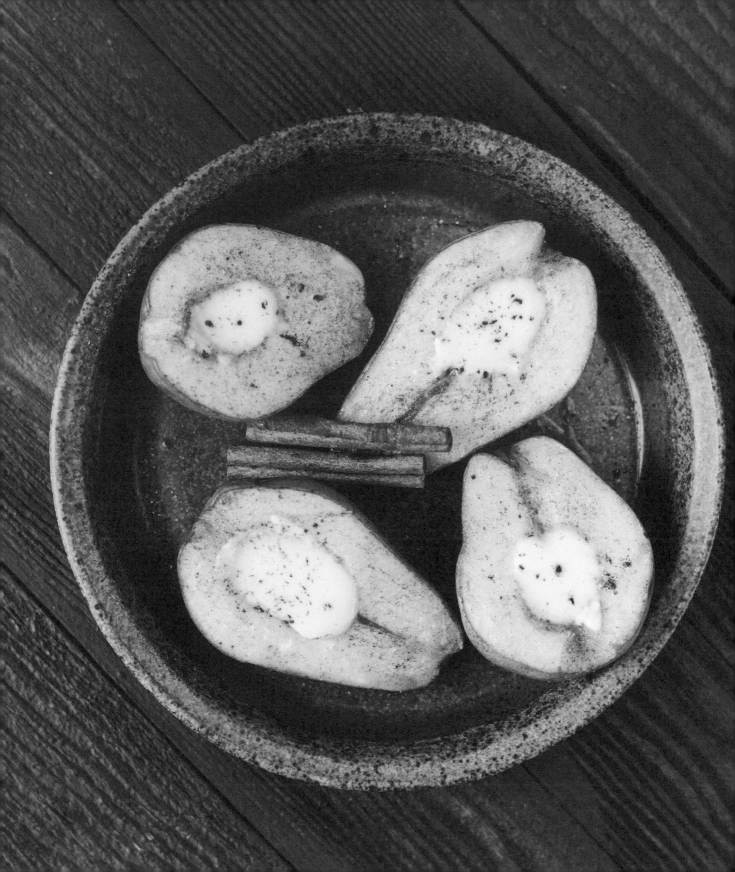

CINNAMON-GINGER BAKED PEARS

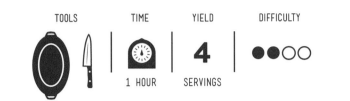

TOOLS   TIME   YIELD   DIFFICULTY

1 HOUR   **4** SERVINGS   ●●○○

2 firm pears, halved and cored

1 tablespoon coconut oil, melted

½ lemon, juiced
(about 1 tablespoon)

⅛ teaspoon ground cinnamon

⅛ teaspoon ground ginger

Pinch of sea salt

2 tablespoons Coconut
Concentrate (page 45)*

1 Preheat the oven to 180°C.

2 Brush the pear halves generously with coconut oil and lemon juice. Mix the cinnamon, ginger and salt in a small bowl and sprinkle evenly over the pears.

3 Place the pears, cut-side up, in a baking dish and bake for 30 minutes, or until soft. Remove from the oven and let cool for a few minutes.

4 Drizzle with coconut concentrate and serve immediately.

*Note: In order to measure the coconut concentrate, it is best to soften it in a warm water bath before use as it is solid at room temperature.

Variation: Feel free to use apples for this recipe, but they may take a bit longer to bake.

Storage: Keeps in the refrigerator for several days.

APPLE-SPICE TEA COOKIES

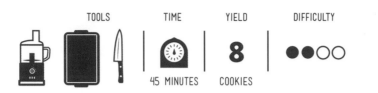

TOOLS	TIME	YIELD	DIFFICULTY
	45 MINUTES	8 COOKIES	●●○○

65 g fine shredded coconut (unsweetened)

2 tablespoons coconut flour

1 apple, peeled, cored and roughly chopped

8 dates, pitted

2 tablespoons coconut oil, plus extra, for greasing

¼ teaspoon ground cinnamon

Pinch of sea salt

1 Preheat the oven to 170°C.

2 Place all ingredients in a food processor and mix until a thick paste forms. Form into 8 round, flat cookies and place on a baking tray greased with a little coconut oil.

3 Bake for 15 minutes, or until barely golden. The cookies will still be a little soft; let cool completely before serving.

Variation: Feel free to use pears for this recipe. You can also use dried figs instead of dates for a less sweet cookie.

Storage: Keeps in the refrigerator for a week. Also freezes well.

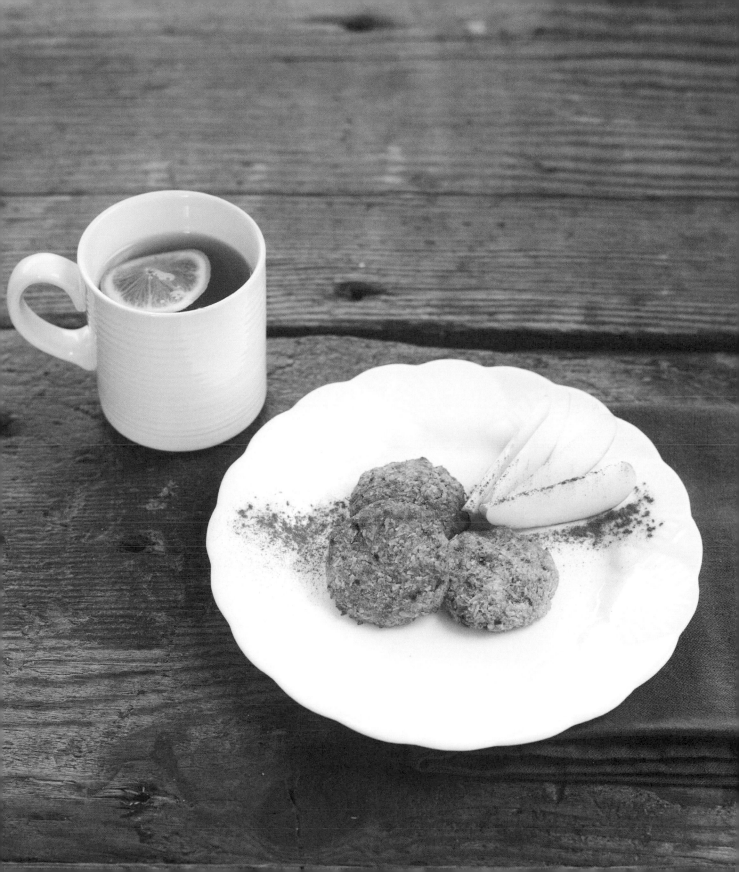

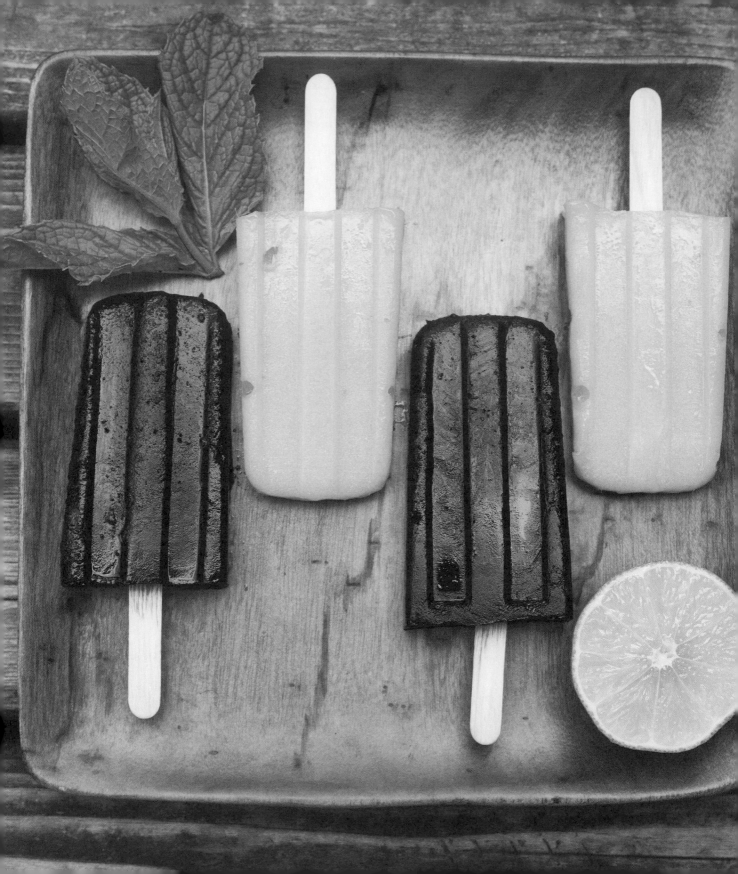

CHERRY-LIME POPSICLES

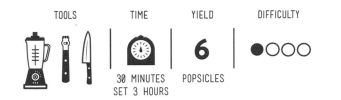

TOOLS   TIME   YIELD   DIFFICULTY

30 MINUTES SET 3 HOURS   **6** POPSICLES

450 g frozen pitted cherries (unsweetened)

125 ml freshly squeezed lime juice (about 12 limes)

½ teaspoon lime zest

¼ teaspoon sea salt

1 Pour the cherries into a shallow dish or bowl and allow them to partially thaw. Put the cherries, lime juice, zest and salt in a blender and blend until smooth.

2 Pour the mixture into popsicle moulds. Freeze completely and serve.

Storage: Keeps in the freezer for a month.

Variation: Substitute frozen berries or pineapple for the cherries.

MANGO-COCONUT POPSICLES

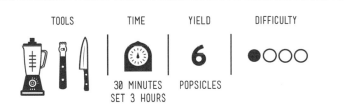

TOOLS   TIME   YIELD   DIFFICULTY

30 MINUTES SET 3 HOURS   **6** POPSICLES

400 g frozen mango

125 ml coconut water

½ teaspoon lemon zest

¼ teaspoon sea salt

1 Put the mango into a shallow dish or bowl and allow to partially thaw. Put the mango, coconut water, zest and salt into a blender and blend until smooth.

2 Pour the mixture into popsicle moulds. Freeze completely and serve.

Storage: Keeps in the freezer for a month.

COCONUT CREAM BOWL

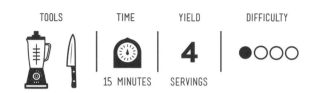

TOOLS | TIME | YIELD | DIFFICULTY

15 MINUTES | 4 SERVINGS | ●○○○

125 ml Coconut Concentrate
  (page 45)*
125 ml filtered water
90 g honey
¼ teaspoon sea salt
30 g raspberries
75 g strawberries, hulled
  and halved
½ kiwi fruit, peeled, halved,
  and cut into thin slices
Pinch of ground cinnamon

1 Place the coconut concentrate, water, honey and salt in a blender and blend for a few seconds, or until thoroughly incorporated. If the mixture is too thick, add more water a tablespoon at a time until desired consistency is reached.

2 Divide the mixture into four cups or bowls and top with the fresh fruit. Add a dusting of cinnamon to each, and serve immediately.

*Note: In order to measure the coconut concentrate, it is best to soften it in a warm water bath before use as it is solid at room temperature.

Variation: Feel free to switch up the fruit and spices—mango and lime zest would be nice, as would pomegranate seeds or blackberries.

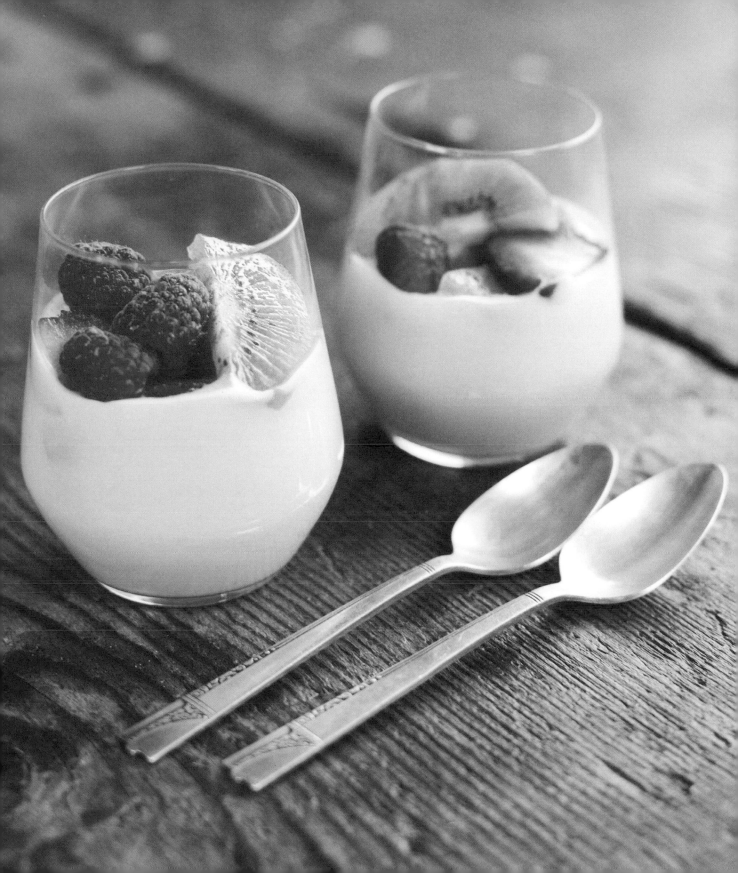

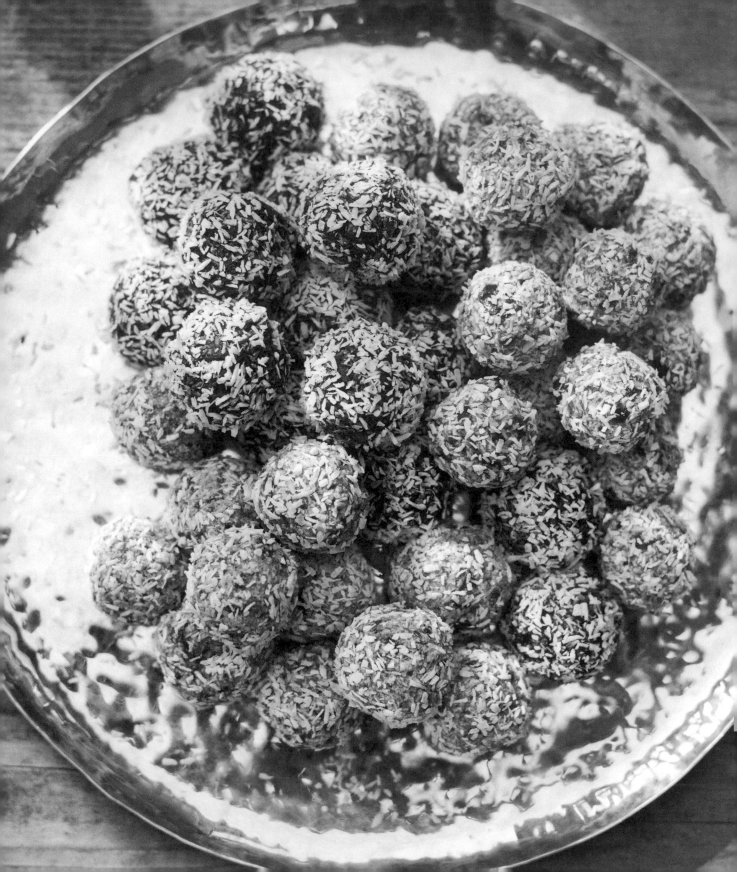

MACAROONS

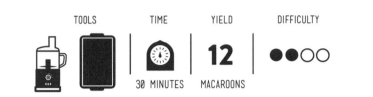

TOOLS	TIME	YIELD	DIFFICULTY
	30 MINUTES	**12** MACAROONS	●●○○

180 g unsweetened desiccated coconut, plus 2 tablespoons, kept separate

225 g dates, pitted and soaked in warm water for 5 minutes

¼ teaspoon alcohol-free vanilla extract (optional)

¼ teaspoon sea salt

1 Preheat the oven to 170°C.

2 Place the 180 g of desiccated coconut, dates, vanilla (if using) and sea salt in a food processor and process until thick and sticky.

3 Place the extra coconut on a small plate. Form the date mixture into little balls, then roll in the coconut for decoration.

4 Place on a greased baking tray and bake for 12 to 15 minutes, or until barely golden.

Lemon Variation: Add 1 tablespoon lemon juice and 1 teaspoon lemon zest to the coconut and date mixture.

Blueberry Variation: Add 115 g of frozen or fresh blueberries to the coconut and date mixture.

Storage: Keeps in the refrigerator for a week. Also freezes well.

RASPBERRY-COCONUT 'CHEESECAKE'

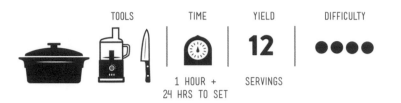

TOOLS	TIME	YIELD	DIFFICULTY
	1 HOUR + 24 HRS TO SET	**12** SERVINGS	●●●●

Crust:

500 g dates, pitted and soaked for 5 minutes in warm water

250 ml coconut oil, melted

35 g coconut flour

30 g unsweetened desiccated coconut

⅛ teaspoon salt

Filling:

380 g Coconut Concentrate (page 45)

340 ml whipped honey

250 ml coconut oil, melted

400 g frozen raspberries

6 tablespoons tapioca starch

1½ teaspoons vanilla extract (optional)

¼ teaspoon sea salt

Thick, unsweetened coconut flakes, for garnish

Fresh raspberries, for garnish

1 Preheat the oven to 170°C.

2 To prepare the crust, strain the dates (discard the water) and place them in a food processor or high-powered blender with the melted coconut oil. Blend for 30 seconds, or until a chunky paste forms. If you are using a standard blender, you may have to stop and scrape the sides; the oil may not completely mix with the dates, but the crust will still turn out fine.

3 Combine the coconut flour, desiccated coconut and salt in a bowl. Add the date paste and mix thoroughly. Place the mixture in the bottom of a 20 cm springform cake tin, pressing it down evenly. Use a small spatula to clean up the top edge around the sides of the pan, where the filling will meet the crust. Bake for 30 to 35 minutes, until the crust browns and hardens a little bit. The texture will still be soft until it finishes cooling. Set aside while you make the filling.

4 Soften the coconut concentrate and honey by placing them in a warm water bath for a few minutes.

5 To make the filling, combine the coconut concentrate, honey, coconut oil and frozen raspberries in a saucepan on low heat. Stir until the raspberries are no longer frozen and the mixture is warm, about 5 minutes. Transfer to a blender and add the tapioca starch, vanilla and salt. Blend on high for about a minute, until completely mixed. Pour carefully on top of the crust.

6 Set in the refrigerator and leave, undisturbed, for at least 12 hours to allow the cake to cool and completely solidify. When it is ready, carefully remove the sides of the cake tin.

7 Decorate the top of the cake with the thick coconut flakes and fresh raspberries.

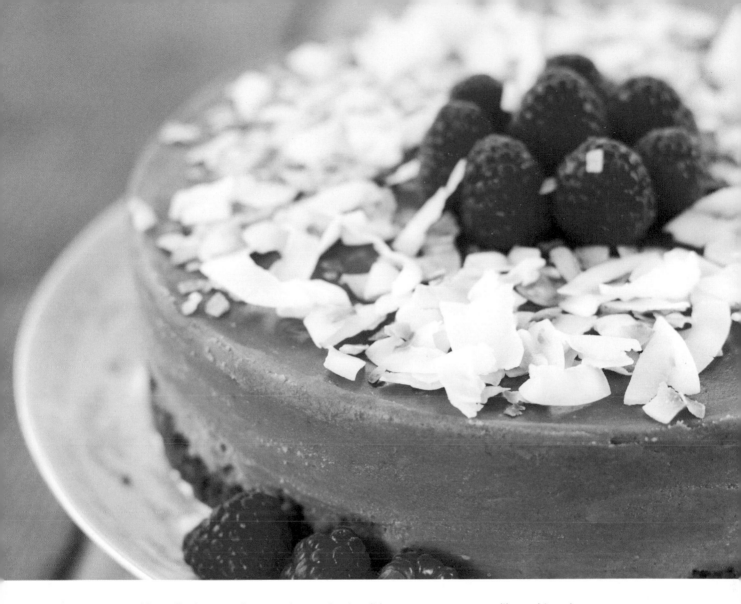

Note: For best results, use a honey that is solid at room temperature, like a whipped product. Make sure you use Coconut Concentrate (page 45), which is not the same as the thick stuff at the top of a tin of coconut milk! If you used the tinned coconut milk, the cake will not set.

Variation: Substitute 465 g of blueberries for the frozen raspberries; for a blueberry-lemon variation, add the juice and zest of 1 lemon.

Storage: Keeps for a week, tightly wrapped, in the refrigerator. Leftover slices can be frozen for later enjoyment!

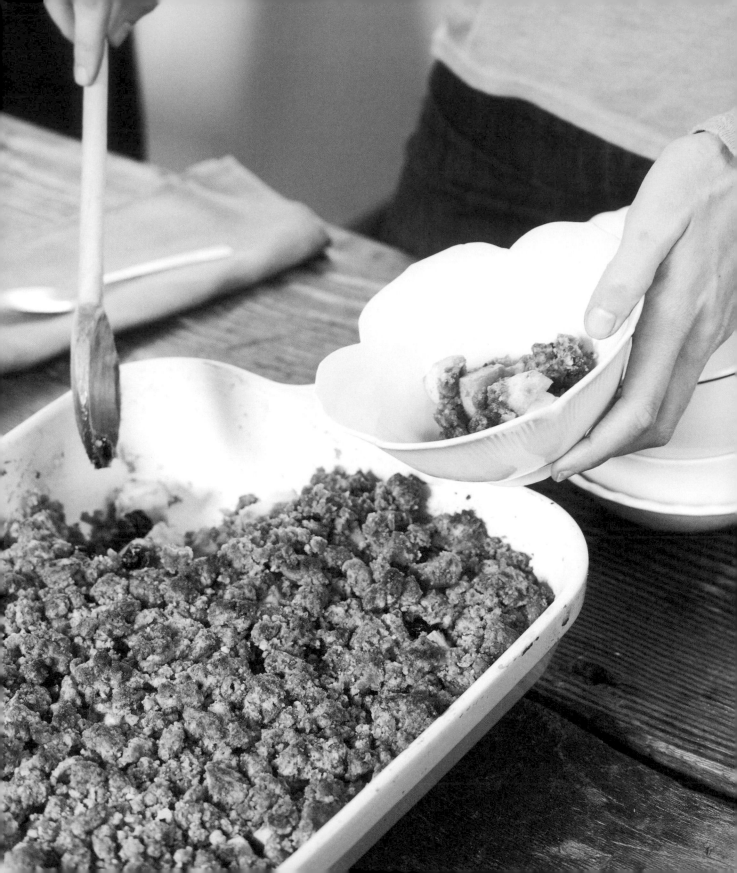

APPLE-CRANBERRY CRUMBLE

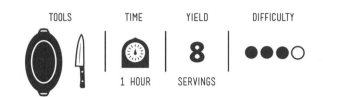

TOOLS | TIME | YIELD | DIFFICULTY

1 HOUR | 8 SERVINGS

Crumble:

375 ml coconut oil, cold

105 g coconut flour

130 g arrowroot flour

120 g coconut sugar

1 teaspoon ground cinnamon

¼ teaspoon sea salt

125 ml cold filtered water

Filling:

6 apples, chopped into
    4 cm pieces

145 g unsweetened dried
    cranberries

60 ml coconut oil, melted

1 lemon, juiced
    (about 2 tablespoons)

1 teaspoon ground cinnamon

1 Preheat the oven to 180°C. If the coconut oil is not already cold, put it in the refrigerator for about 10 minutes to chill.

2 In a large bowl, combine the coconut flour, arrowroot flour, coconut sugar, cinnamon and salt. Using a pastry cutter, cut in the coconut oil until you have pea-size lumps. Sprinkle in the cold water and gently mix—you want the crumble topping to stay chunky and not turn into dough. Set aside.

3 In another large bowl, combine the apples, cranberries, coconut oil, lemon juice and cinnamon. Mix until well combined. Place in a 23 x 33 cm baking dish and cover with the crumble topping.

4 Bake for 40 minutes, until lightly browned on top. Remove from the oven, let cool a little bit and serve warm.

Variation: Feel free to use pears instead of apples, or raisins instead of cranberries.

Storage: Keeps in the refrigerator for several days; also freezes well.

PEAR-CARAMEL PIE

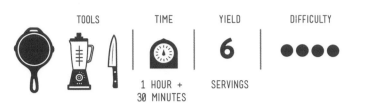

TOOLS	TIME	YIELD	DIFFICULTY
	1 HOUR + 30 MINUTES	**6** SERVINGS	●●●●

Crust:

175 ml coconut oil, cold

105 g coconut flour

130 g arrowroot flour

¼ teaspoon sea salt

125 ml cold filtered water

1 tablespoon coconut oil, melted

Filling:

3 tablespoons coconut oil

4 tablespoons coconut sugar

1 teaspoon ground cinnamon

½ teaspoon sea salt

1 teaspoon alcohol-free vanilla (optional)

4 firm pears

1 Preheat the oven to 170°C. If the coconut oil for the crust is not already cold, put it in the refrigerator for about 10 minutes to chill.

2 Halve and core all of the pears, setting one aside and slicing the rest into thin, 5 mm slices.

3 In a bowl, combine the coconut flour, arrowroot flour and salt. Using a pastry cutter, cut in the coconut oil until you have pea-size lumps. Add the cold water and mix. It will still be crumbly—not like regular dough! Don't overmix.

4 Place the mixture into a deep 23 cm pie dish. Using your fingers, spread it evenly across the bottom and up the sides. Prick some holes in the bottom of the crust with a fork, then brush the crust with the melted coconut oil. Bake for 15 minutes, until the crust browns. The texture will be soft as it finishes cooling. Set aside while you make the filling.

5 Heat the 3 tablespoons coconut oil and sugar for the filling in a medium saucepan. Cook for about 10 minutes, stirring until the sugar is caramelised and golden brown (don't be alarmed if it separates from the oil—this is normal). Pour the mixture into a bowl to cool a little bit before placing into a blender with the cinnamon, salt, vanilla (if using) and the pear that was cored but left unsliced. Blend on high until thoroughly mixed. Place the caramel sauce in a bowl and set aside.

6 Increase the oven temperature to 180°C. Arrange the pear slices in a pinwheel, overlapping them, on top of the baked crust. Pour the caramel sauce evenly over the top; bake for 35 minutes, or until the crust is golden brown and the sauce is bubbling. Let cool for a few minutes and serve warm.

Variation: Feel free to use apples instead of pears here, although they may take longer to bake. You may also slice the fruit into chunks instead of making the pinwheel design.

Storage: Keeps in the refrigerator for several days; also freezes well.

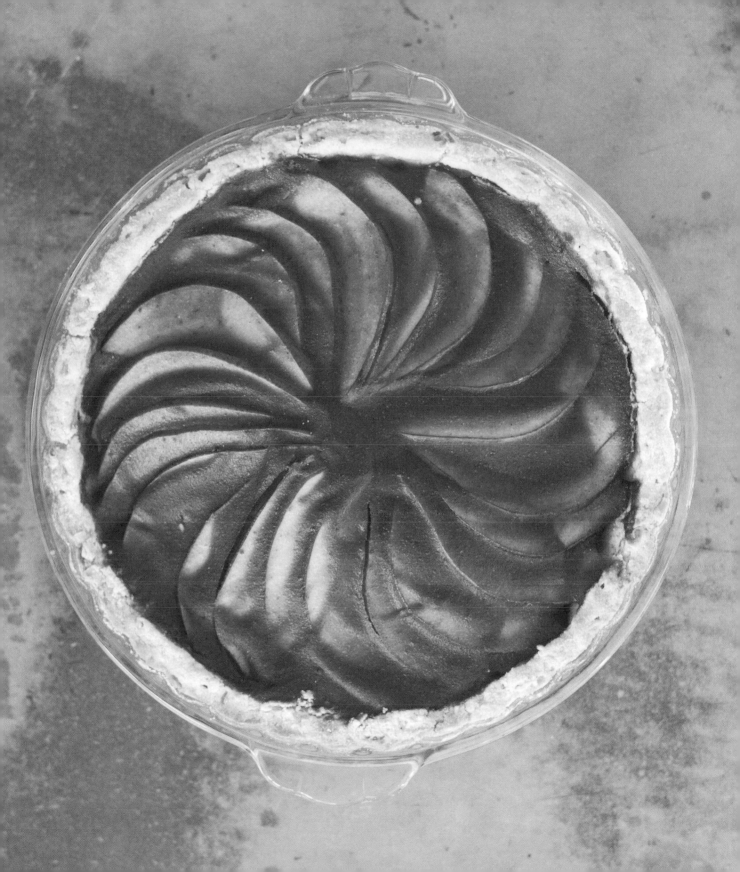

ONLINE RESOURCES

autoimmune-paleo.com – My website, where I share recipes as well as articles about diet and autoimmunity.

balancedbites.com – A great resource by Diane Sanfilippo, author of *Practical Paleo*. Lots of information for those looking into ancestral nutrition or paleo, with great ideas and recipes.

chriskresser.com – One of the best sources for scientific information about ancestral nutrition.

terrywahls.com – A resource for information on multiple sclerosis and diet by Terry Wahls, MD, who has put her own disease into remission using similar principles.

thepaleomom.com – The website of Sarah Ballantyne, PhD, author of *The Paleo Approach* and *The Paleo Approach Cookbook*. Her site is the best resource on the internet for information about the Autoimmune Protocol; it also contains many wonderful recipes.

whole9life.com - A great resource for those looking to try the Autoimmune Protocol in conjunction with Whole 30, a month-long clean-eating challenge lead by Dallas and Melissa Hartwig.

Finding A Practitioner

functionalmedicine.org – The website of the Institute for Functional Medicine, where you can find a doctor who specialises in the functional treatment of autoimmune disease.

primaldocs.com – A resource to find a doctor or health care practitioner who uses an ancestral approach to health and nutrition.

http://acnem.org – The Australasian College of Nutritional and Environmental Medicine.

http://mindd.org – MINDD Foundation

Hashimoto's Disease

facebook.com/groups/EPDiet411/ - A wonderful support group for those interested in the elimination/provocation diet run by Kirsten Liston.

hashimotoshealing.com – Excellent information on the functional treatment of Hashimoto's disease by Marc Ryan, L.Ac.

thyroidbook.com – Dr. Datis Kharrazian's website, which has information about functional medicine and Hashimoto's disease.

Autoimmune Protocol Patient Blogs

acleanplate.com – Written by Christina Feindel, a patient advocate with Hashimoto's—this site has lots of great allergen-free recipes.

alt-ternativeautoimmune.blogspot.com – A blog by Angela Alt, who has used the protocol to heal from multiple autoimmune diseases. Angela shares recipes as well as the emotional side of healing from autoimmunity.

nutrisclerosis.com – An inspiring blog about the Autoimmune Protocol written by a woman with multiple sclerosis, Whitney Gray.

paleoparents.com – An excellent blog about paleo, parenting and the Autoimmune Protocol, written by Stacy Toth and Matthew McCarry.

phoenixhelix.com – A blog written by Eileen Laird, a woman who has used the protocol to heal her rheumatoid arthritis.

somerealitybites.com - A blog about living, learning and thriving with Hashimoto's disease written by Susan Vennerholm.

Sourcing Food

ewg.org/foodnews – 'Dirty dozen' guide to which fruits and vegetables contain the highest amounts of pesticides.

farmersmarkets.org.au/markets

farmersmarkets.org.nz

sustainabletable.org.au

australianorganicdirectory.com.au

farma.org.uk

Bone Broth

balancedbites.com/2011/04/easy-recipe-mineral-rich-bone-broth.html

westonaprice.org/food-features/broth-is-beautiful

Fermented Beverages

culturesforhealth.com

kombuchakamp.com

Fermented Vegetables

culturesforhealth.com

wildfermentation.com

BOOKS FOR CONTINUING EDUCATION

Digestive Health with Real Food: A Practical Guide to an Anti-Inflammatory, Nutrient-Dense Diet for IBS and Other Digestive Issues, by Aglaee Jacob

It Starts With Food: Discover the Whole30 and Change Your Life in Unexpected Ways by Dallas and Melissa Hartwig

Hashimoto's Thyroiditis: Lifestyle Interventions for Treating the Root Cause, by Izabella Wentz

Practical Paleo: A Customized Approach to Health and a Whole-Foods Lifestyle, by Diane Sanfilippo

The Autoimmune Paleo Breakthrough: A Revolutionary Protocol to Rapidly Decrease Inflammation and Balance Your Immune System, by Anne Angelone

The Hidden Plague: A Field Guide For Surviving and Overcoming Hidradenitis Suppurativa, by Tara Grant

The Paleo Approach: Reverse Autoimmune Disease, Heal Your Body, by Sarah Ballantyne

The Paleo Approach Cookbook: A Detailed Guide to Heal Your Body and Nourish Your Soul, by Sarah Ballantyne

The Paleo Solution: The Original Human Diet, by Robb Wolf

Why Do I Still Have Thyroid Symptoms When My Lab Tests Are Normal? A Revolutionary Breakthrough in Understanding Hashimoto's Disease and Hypothyroidism, by Datis Kharrazian

Why Isn't My Brain Working: A Revolutionary Understanding of Brain Decline and Effective Strategies to Recover Your Brain's Health, by Datis Kharrazian

REFERENCES

1. 'Autoimmune Statistics', American Autoimmune Related Diseases Association, Inc, accessed September 15, 2013, http://www.aarda.org/autoimmune-information/autoimmune-statistics.

2. Sarah Ballantyne, *The Paleo Approach: Reverse Autoimmune Disease, Heal Your Body* (Las Vegas: Victory Belt, 2013), 53-57

3. Datis Kharrazian, *Why Do I Still Have Thyroid Symptoms? When My Lab Tests Are Normal: A Revolutionary Breakthrough in Understanding Hashimoto's Disease and Hypothyroidism* (Carlsbad: Elephant Press, 2010), 123-124

4. Robb Wolf, *The Paleo Solution: The Original Human Diet* (Las Vegas: Victory Belt, 2010), 201

5. Robb Wolf, *The Paleo Solution: The Original Human Diet* (Las Vegas: Victory Belt, 2010), 197-210

6. Sarah Ballantyne, *The Paleo Approach: Reverse Autoimmune Disease, Heal Your Body* (Las Vegas: Victory Belt, 2013), 185-186

7. Sarah Ballantyne, *The Paleo Approach: Reverse Autoimmune Disease, Heal Your Body* (Las Vegas: Victory Belt, 2013), 185-235

8. Sarah Ballantyne, *The Paleo Approach: Reverse Autoimmune Disease, Heal Your Body* (Las Vegas: Victory Belt, 2013), 53-57

9. Datis Kharrazian, *Why Do I Still Have Thyroid Symptoms? When My Lab Tests Are Normal: A Revolutionary Breakthrough in Understanding Hashimoto's Disease and Hypothyroidism* (Carlsbad: Elephant Press, 2010), 123

10. Aglaee Jacob, *Digestive Health with REAL Food: A Practical Guide to an Anti-Inflammatory, Nutrient Dense Diet for IBS and Other Digestive Issues* (Bend: Paleo Media group, 2013), 16-18

11. Sarah Ballantyne, *The Paleo Approach: Reverse Autoimmune Disease, Heal Your Body* (Las Vegas: Victory Belt, 2013), 264

12. Elson M. Haas, *Staying Healthy With Nutrition, The Complete Guide to Diet and Nutritional Medicine* (New York: Ten Speed Press, 2006), 83-248

ABOUT THE AUTHOR

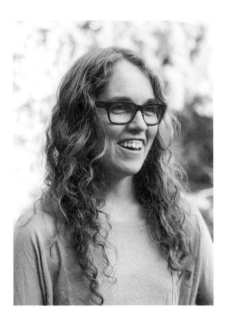

Mickey Trescott lives in the Willamette Valley, Oregon, with her crafty husband, their cat, Savannah, and an assortment of horses, ducks, chickens and goats. She practices nutritional therapy and cooks privately for local families in addition to blogging and obsessively knitting socks in her spare time. After recovering from her own struggle with both Coeliac and Hashimoto's disease, adrenal fatigue and multiple vitamin deficiencies, Mickey started to blog about her experiences at autoimmune-paleo.com. Her hope is to give others on a similar path a resource to find information—and to help them realise that they are not alone in their struggles. She also aims to provide a supportive environment for those seeking better health in the face of autoimmunity.

ABOUT THE PHOTOGRAPHER

Hailing from the Pacific Northwest, Kyle Johnson creates images that are intriguing and classically executed. Whether it's portrait or travel work, Kyle's aesthetic pairs textured natural settings with a distinct photographic perspective. He has shot for publications like *The New York Times Magazine, Wallpaper*, *Sunset, Kinfolk, Popular Mechanics* and more.

GRATITUDE

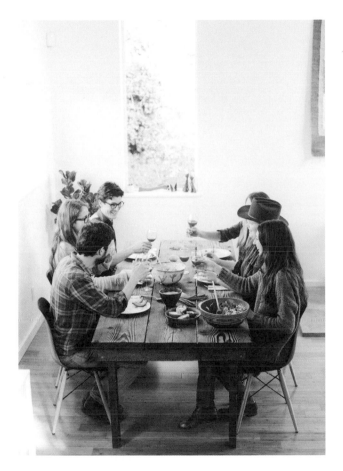

Thank you to all who have supported me in the journey of writing my first cookbook! It has been an incredible experience, and I would not have been able to do it without the support of many people.

Thank you to my friends, family, and blog readers who supported the crowd-funding campaign to produce this book—I am grateful for your contributions!

Thank you to Mary Cloos for the last-minute proof-read. Thank you to Edward and Nancy at Star Print Brokers, for graciously answering all of my questions and making self-publishing a breeze. Thank you to Lisa and Jeffrey, for your patience and support through this process.

Thank you to Devyn Perez, Eric Elliott, Jane Thomas, Katie Sullivan, Felix Madrid, Rob Miller, Susan Vennerholm, Melanie Penney, and Jenny Littlefield for helping test recipes and assisting me on photo-shoot days.

Thank you to Crown S. Ranch and Olsen Farms for sustainably raising the quality meat I used to develop my recipes.

Thank you to Kyle Johnson, Brenna Rose Miller and Chris Black for being an incredible team and enabling me to produce such a high-quality book.

Thank you to my parents, Rose and Brian, for their endless love and support and for always encouraging me to follow my dreams.

Lastly, thank you to my husband Noah, who encouraged me to write this book in the first place—I am sorry you didn't know what you were getting yourself into! (But I hope the food was worth it ...)

INDEX

Published in 2016 by Murdoch Books, an imprint of Allen & Unwin
First published in 2014 by Trescott LLC

Murdoch Books Australia
83 Alexander Street
Crows Nest NSW 2065
Phone: +61 (0) 2 8425 0100
Fax: +61 (0) 2 9906 2218
murdochbooks.com.au
info@murdochbooks.com.au

Murdoch Books UK
Erico House, 6th Floor
93–99 Upper Richmond Road
Putney, London SW15 2TG
Phone: +44 (0) 20 8785 5995
murdochbooks.co.uk
info@murdochbooks.co.uk

For Corporate Orders & Custom Publishing contact
Noel Hammond, National Business Development Manager, Murdoch Books Australia

Publisher: Corinne Roberts
Photography: Kyle Johnson, www.kjphotos.com
Styling: Brenna Rose Designs, www.brennarosedesigns.com
Design: Chris Black, www.theblackresidence.com
Editorial manager: Katie Bosher
Production manager: Alex Gonzalez

A cataloguing-in-publication entry is available from the catalogue of the National Library of Australia at nla.gov.au.

ISBN 978 1 74336 808 4 Australia
ISBN 978 1 74336 819 0 UK

A catalogue record for this book is available from the British Library.

Disclaimer: The content presented in this book is meant for inspiration and informational purposes only. The purchaser of this book understands that the author is not a medical professional, and the information contained within this book is not intended to replace medical advice or meant to be relied upon to treat, cure, or prevent any disease, illness, or medical condition. It is understood that you will seek full medical clearance by a licensed physician before making any changes mentioned in this book. The author and publisher claim no responsibility to any person or entity for any liability, loss, or damage caused or alleged to be caused directly or indirectly as a result of the use, application, or interpretation of the material in this book.

Colour reproduction by Splitting Image Colour Studio Pty Ltd, Clayton, Victoria
Printed by 1010 Printing International Limited, China

OVEN GUIDE: You may find cooking times vary depending on the oven you are using. For fan-forced ovens, as a general rule, set the oven temperature to 20°C (35°F) lower than indicated in the recipe.

MEASURES GUIDE: We have used 15 ml tablespoon (3 teaspoon) measures.